LUNG FUNCTION TESTS
A guide to their interpretation

Lung Function Tests

A guide to their interpretation

Dr William JM Kinnear
University Hospital, Nottingham

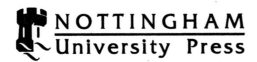

NOTTINGHAM University Press

Nottingham University Press
Manor Farm, Main Street
Thrumpton, Nottingham, NG11 0AX, UK

NOTTINGHAM

First published 1997
Reprinted 1999
Second reprint 2002
© Dr William JM Kinnear

British Library Cataloguing in Publication Data
A catalogue record for this book is available from the British Library

ISBN   1-897676-80-8

Typeset by Nottingham University Press, Nottingham
Digitally reproduced by Lightning Source

PREFACE

Every doctor training to be a specialist in respiratory medicine needs to know how to interpret lung function tests, and they are likely to be involved at some stage in writing formal reports on the results of such tests. The primary aim of this book is to help them in this task. However, the person in the best position to interpret a set of lung function tests is often the clinician who sits with the patient in front of them, chest x-rays and scans at hand. It follows from this that any doctor who regularly requests lung function tests, or who sees patients who have had such tests performed, should know how to interpret them. I hope therefore that this book is accessible enough also to be of use to those who are not specialists in respiratory medicine.

Lung function tests now feature in many post-graduate examinations. All the tests likely to be encountered in this context are covered and with this in mind, I have aimed to keep this volume sufficiently short and simple so that it will be a useful aid to revision.

Lung function tests covered

In the title of this book, by "lung function tests" I really mean "commonly-used lung function tests". Spirometry, flow volume loops, lung volumes and carbon monoxide transfer are all covered in some detail, with shorter sections on blood gases and exercise testing. I acknowledge that the inclusion of tests of respiratory muscle function may appear rather idiosyncratic to some, reflecting my own interest in this expanding field. I have not devoted any space to the sorts of tests (lung compliance, nitrogen washout, nitric oxide transfer, control of breathing etc etc) which are usually only performed by larger laboratories.

What this book is not

This is not a technical manual - I have assumed that you are presented with lung function data the quality of which you can rely on. The practical details of performing tests, calibration and quality control are dealt with admirably in other texts.

Neither is this a physiology textbook. Clearly an understanding of respiratory physiology is central to the ability to interpret lung function tests, but there are already many excellent books on this subject. Reading books on respiratory physiology greatly expands the knowledge of the reader, but often does little to empower them to actually interpret a set of lung function data. The aim of this book is to focus on this thought process, and I have not included much in the way of technical details or respiratory physiology in order to avoid clouding my main aim.

Further reading

The text of this book contains a scant sprinkling of references, the purpose of which is to give the reader a lead into the relevant literature. It is not intended to be an exhaustive source of references, which can be found in the texts listed in the bibliography. These should be consulted for more detail on individual tests and diseases, and for the less commonly used tests which I do not cover.

LIST OF ABREVIATIONS

ARTP	Association of Respiratory Technicians and Physiologists
AT	anaerobic threshold
ATS	American Thoracic Society
BMI	body mass index
bpm	beats per minute
BTS	British Thoracic Society
cm	centimetre
cmH₂O	centimetre of water
CO	carbon monoxide
COAD	chronic obstructive airways disease
CXR	chest X-ray
dl	decilitre
ERS	European Respiratory Society
FEV1	forced expiratory volume in one second
FiO₂	inspired fractional concentration of oxygen
FRC	functional residual capacity
FV	flow-volume
FVC	forced vital capacity
Hb	haemoglobin
IVC	inspiratory vital capacity
KCO	tranfer coefficient for carbon monoxide
kg	kilogram
kPa	kilopascal
L	litre
m	metre
mg	milligram
MEP	maximum expiratory pressure
min	minute
MIP	maximum inspiratory pressure
mmHg	millimetres of mercury
ml	millilitre
nmol	nanomole
PaCO₂	arterial partial pressure of carbon dioxide
PaO₂	arterial partial pressure of oxygen
PEFR	peak expiratory flow rate
RSD	residual standard deviation
RV	residual volume
RVC	relaxed vital capacity
s	second
SNIP	maximal sniff nasal pressure
SD	standard deviation
SGaw	specific airways conductance
SI	systeme internationale
SR	standardised residual
TGV	thoracic gas volume
TLC	total lung capacity
TLCO	transfer factor for carbon monoxide
VA	alveolar volume
VEmax	maximum ventilation
VO₂max	maximum oxygen uptake
VC	vital capacity
yrs	years

vii

For Sue, Anne and Katie

CONTENTS

1: INTRODUCTION

DATA COLLECTION

This book is about how to interpret lung function tests. It is not about how to perform the tests themselves, this being the domain of the technician rather than the doctor who is reporting the tests. I have assumed that you are able to use the test equipment competently (for example, a simple spirometer in the out-patient clinic) or that you have faith in the skill of your technicians, and that you can therefore rely on the quality of the data you are presented with.

I have also assumed that in the calculation of predicted values, equations suitable for that patient (taking account of ethnic origin, using arm span instead of height in the presence of spinal deformity, etc), on that test equipment, have been used.

PRESENTATION OF RESULTS

With the introduction of computers into the lung function laboratory, there is a trend towards the inclusion of an increasing number of parameters in the printed results which are produced. For example, Figure 1.1 shows a simple volume-time trace, such as that commonly recorded with a Vitalograph bellows spirometer:

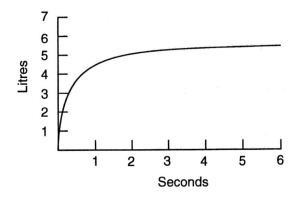

Figure 1.1

Some of the measurements that can be made on, or derived from, such a trace are listed below. There are quite a few more!

FVC

FEV .5

FEV 1

FEV 2

FEV 3

FEF 75 (Forced expiratory flow at 75% FVC)

FEF 50

FEF 25

FEF 25-75 (Mean mid-expiratory flow)

FMFT (Forced mid-expiratory flow time)

FEF 0.2-1.2 (Forced expiratory flow from 0.2 to 1.2 L)

PEFR

FEV1/FVC%

MTT (Mean transit time)

FET (Forced expiratory time)

FETPEF (Forced expiratory time at PEFR)

FEVPEF (Forced expiratory volume at PEFR)

Alpha-1 75 (First moment to 75% FVC)

MR 75 (Moment ratio to 75% FVC)

Many of these options are available on modern computerised systems, and it is tempting to include many of them in the print-out. The result is a long list, which is pretty indigestible. Moreover, the more parameters that are presented, the higher the chances of throwing up a false positive[1].

Most of these data you do not use in forming your interpretation, and after a time you train yourself so that you only consciously "see" the data you wish to use, as if a blanking template were placed over the full print-out:

FVC	5.5 litres
FEV .5	
FEV 1	4.3 litres
FEV 2	
FEV 3	
FEF 75	
FEF 50	
FEF 25	
FEF 25-75	
FMFT	
FEF 0.2-1.2	
PEFR	
FEV1/FVC%	78%
MTT	
FET	
FETPEF	
FEVPEF	
Alpha-1 75	
MR 75	

For clinical purposes, these three parameters can be used to derive almost all the useful information contained in the volume-time trace. FVC is the Forced Vital Capacity, which is used as an indication of the size of the lungs. FEV1 is the volume expired in the first second (Forced Expiratory Volume in 1 second), and the ratio of this to FVC reflects the resistance of the airways. (More on this later.)

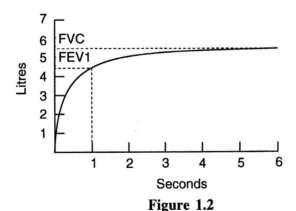

Figure 1.2

Those of you who have worked in different hospitals with different lung function test print-outs will know that it takes a while to "get your eye in" for each different system, as you have to re-learn a way of scanning the data, with a sub-conscious new blanking-out pattern. I have tried to keep the examples in this book as simple as possible, using the same general format throughout. (If you are designing a print-out, try and include only the data you actually use. There will be rare occasions when you want some additional information, for example a mean mid-expiratory flow rate, but you can usually ask for this to be retrieved from stored data.)

PATIENT 1.01

Sex:	Male	Height (m):	1.76
Age (yrs):	18	Weight (kg):	62
Tobacco:	Non-smoker	BMI (kg/m²):	20

	Measured	% Predicted
Spirometry:		
FEV (L)	4.3	94
VC (L)	5.5	103
FEV1/VC(%)	78	93

Another column will appear in the next chapter, and there will be additional results to add as we move on to cover different lung function tests.

PHILOSOPHY OF INTERPRETATION

In interpreting lung function data, we recognise patterns of abnormality which fit certain clinical scenarios. Part of the art of this process is learning whether or not to ignore parts of the picture which do not quite fit the general pattern. Does an isolated abnormality of only one lung volume mean anything of any clinical significance? It is worth remembering that if a large number of tests are performed often enough in normal subjects, from time to time one will lie outside the normal range. Beware of over-interpretation.

Your aim in interpreting a set of lung function tests should be to derive some information which is of clinical value. This point is perhaps easiest to demonstrate when we write down our opinion in a formal report.

THE FORMAL REPORT

When asked to give a written report, it is a relatively easy task just to summarise the lung function data and put:

> *"Mild restrictive defect; normal gas transfer".*

In some instances this will suffice, and this is the usual response of someone presented with a pile of lung function print-outs who is either uninterested or pressed for time. However, it is often possible to be much more helpful to the clinician who requested the tests, along the lines of:

> *"Mild restrictive defect on the basis of slightly low TLC, but this is unlikely to explain the patient's breathlessness, particularly since the carbon monoxide transfer factor is normal".*

Try to encourage the clinician who will read your report to interpret the data and consider the report within the clinical context. A patient referred with the clinical information on the request form given as "COAD - any reversibility ?" might have lung function data which prompt you to write:

> *"Restrictive defect with no evidence of airflow obstruction. High KCO with normal TLCO could be explained by extra-pulmonary restriction. Is there any evidence of pleural disease, muscle weakness or thoracic deformity?"*

Lung function tests are seldom diagnostic, but the patterns of abnormality often fit with a fairly small group of diseases in the direction of which the clinician can be pointed. They may well have clinical information available which makes your suggestion of, for example, fibrosing alveolitis very unlikely, but you may point to diagnoses that they had not previously considered. Try not to over-interpret, be as helpful as possible, suggest further tests which might be of value, and remember that the person requesting the tests will have lots of additional information available which they can be encouraged to match to your report.

COMPUTER INTERPRETATION

Interpreting lung function data is an art, the thought processes behind which are complex. A computer cannot, as yet, give a report along the lines of the fuller reports given in the previous section of this chapter. Computer algorithms exist which can detect patterns within the data, but they do not take account of the clinical information available and do not at present generate reports which are of much value to clinicians. A couple of references may be of interest to those stimulated to explore this topic further[2,3].

SUMMARY

☞ If you perform lots of lung function tests on a normal individual, some of the results may lie outside the normal range.

☞ An isolated abnormal lung function test result should be interpreted with caution.

☞ Lung function tests are seldom diagnostic, but do fall into a number of patterns of abnormality.

☞ In reporting lung function tests, we can see if the pattern of abnormality fits the clinical picture, suggest alternative diagnoses for the clinician to consider, and recommend further tests.

☞ Humans are better at this than computers (at the moment).

REFERENCES

1.   Vedal S, Crapo RO. False positive rates of multiple pulmonary function tests in healthy subjects. *Bull Eur Physiopathol Respir* 1983;**19**:263–266.

2.   Ellis JH, Perera SP, Levin DC. A computer program for calculation and interpretation of pulmonary function studies. *Chest* 1975;**68**:209–213.

3.   Heise D, Kroker P, Mailander A. An expert system for synoptic interpretation of lung function tests. *Lung* 1990; suppl:1193–1200.

2: "WITHIN NORMAL LIMITS"

NORMAL OR ABNORMAL?

The first stage in the process of interpreting a set of lung function tests such as those from Patient 2.01 is to decide whether or not the results are abnormal.

PATIENT 2.01

Sex:	Male	Height (m):	1.65
Age (yrs):	50	Weight (kg):	74
Tobacco:	Ex-smoker	BMI (kg/m²):	27

	Measured	*% Predicted*
Spirometry:		
FEV1 (L)	2.35	74
VC (L)	2.92	76
FEV1/VC (%)	80	103
Lung Volumes: (Helium dilution)		
RV (L)	1.41	69
FRC (L)	2.25	70
TLC (L)	5.14	84

At this stage we won't worry too much about what the volumes mean, but to refresh your memory here are how they are derived from classical spirograms:

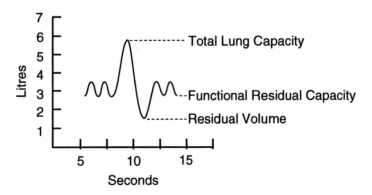

Figure 2.1

Clearly the FEV1/VC at 103% predicted is fine, and TLC is probably not significantly reduced, but what about the other volumes? Traditionally, 80% predicted has often been taken as the cut-off for normality, but this has little scientific basis. (Electrolyte results don't come back from the laboratory as Sodium 67%, Potassium 203%, Urea 145%, Creatinine 181%). Why don't we have a normal range for each parameter, like Sodium (119-131 mmol/L) ? Well, most lung volumes vary with age and height or both, so we need to calculate a normal range for each patient.

Here are the same results with the normal range included:

PATIENT 2.01

	Measured	*% Predicted*	*Normal Range*
Spirometry:			
FEV1(L)	2.35	75	2.31-3.99
VC (L)	2.92	76	2.86-4.86
FEV1/VC (%)	80	103	66-90
Lung Volumes: (Helium dilution)			
RV (L)	1.41	69	1.36-2.70
FRC (L)	2.25	70	2.23-4.21
TLC (L)	5.14	84	4.96-7.26

As you can see by comparing the first column with the third, all the measured results lie within the normal range, although as the results are presented it is a bit tedious having to skip across the page to compare each volume with its normal range. You should conclude *"Within normal limits"*.

If we express these the normal ranges for this patient as percent predicted, we obtain the following values:

	Normal Range *(% Predicted)*
Spirometry:	
FEV1	73-127
VC	74-126
FEV1/VC	85-115
Lung Volumes: (Helium dilution)	
RV	67-133
FRC	69-131
TLC	81-119

The lower limits of 'normality' range from 85% for FEV1/VC to 67% for RV, so a single percentage value for the lower limit of normality is inappropriate for all tests.

As we noted above, comparing measured values to the normal range is rather more laborious than looking at the percent predicted values. Is there an alternative to percent predicted which is as easy to use but more reliably delineates normality from abnormality? The normal range is defined as follows:

Predicted value - (1.64 x RSD) to Predicted value + (1.64 x RSD)

where RSD is the Residual Standard Deviation from the equation used to calculate the predicted value. The RSD is an index of the scatter of the values obtained in the normal population from which the equation is drawn, so the larger the RSD the wider the normal range. This concept should be familiar from the first day of statistics courses and normal distributions (Figure 2.2).

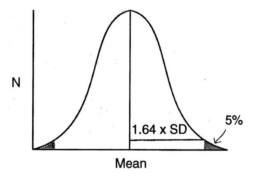

Figure 2.2

For TLC the predicted value is related to height, shown here together with the upper and lower limits of the normal range:

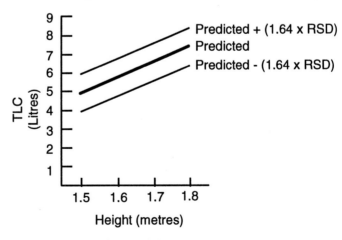

Figure 2.3

The value of 1.64 gives the 90% confidence interval for normality, 1.96 gives the 95% confidence interval[1]. There is incomplete agreement on which value should be used, but 1.64 seems to be more generally favoured and this is the value I have chosen. (One advantage of 1.96 is that 2.00 could be used as an approximation which is much easier to remember.)

In order to decide whether a result is abnormal, why don't we look to see how far the measured result is from the predicted, and then compare this difference to the RSD? If the difference between measured and predicted is more than 1.64 x the RSD, the result is outside the normal range. (Remember that we defined the normal range as predicted +/- (1.64 x RSD)).

In example 2.1 above, the predicted value (taken from the ERS equations) for TLC is 6.10 L[2]. The RSD for TLC in males in these equations is 0.70. If our measurements had yielded a TLC of 4.95 L, at the lower limit of the normal range, subtracting the predicted from the measured value would give -1.15 (4.95 minus 6.10) L. Dividing this difference by the RSD gives exactly -1.64 (-1.15 divided by 0.70), which is hardly surprising since this is how we defined the normal range in the first place:

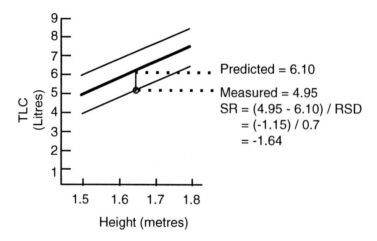

Figure 2.4

The calculation we have just performed is called the Standardised Residual[3], or SR:

$$SR = (Measured\ value - Predicted\ value)\ /\ RSD$$

If the SR is less than -1.64 then the measured value is too low:

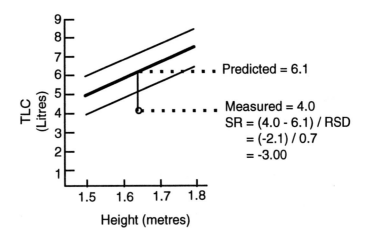

Figure 2.5

If the SR is greater than +1.64 then the measured value is too high:

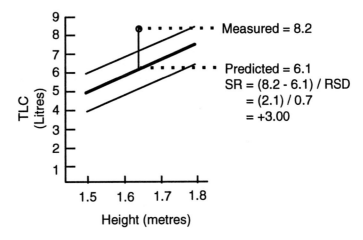

Figure 2.6

Clearly if the measured and predicted values are identical, the SR will be zero:

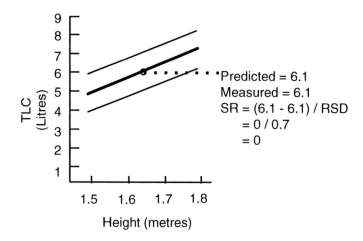

Figure 2.7

From this point onwards, all measurements will be given with their SRs. For legibility, the predicted value and normal range will be omitted, since they do not give any additional information. As yet, SRs are included in the print-outs of only a few lung function testing systems, so I shall still give the percent predicted. Nevertheless, try to get used to looking at the SRs. You may notice that in some of the examples the SR is less negative than -1.64 (i.e. the measured value is not below the lower limit of normality) even although the percent predicted is less than 80%. (Even more of the values less than 80% predicted would be within the normal range if we used -1.96 x RSD as the lower limit of normality).

If we take SRs as the gold standard, spuriously "abnormal" results with percent predicted values of <80% or >120% but normal SRs are quite common for RV and KCO; if you only rely on the percent predicted approach, beware of overinterpretation of an isolated abnormality of either.

Patient 2.02 illustrates the format in which most of the examples in the remainder of this book will be presented. Examine the results and decide whether the results are normal or not. All you need to do is scan down the SR column looking for absolute values of more than 1.64. (Absolute means ignoring the sign, so -1.64 and +1.64 both have absolute values of 1.64).

PATIENT 2.02

Sex:	Female	Height (m):	1.74
Age (yrs):	57	Weight (kg):	78
Tobacco:	Non-smoker	BMI (kg/m²):	26

	Measured	*% Predicted*	*SR*
Spirometry:			
FEV1 (L)	3.00	105	+0.40
VC (L)	3.60	108	+0.61
FEV1/VC (%)	83	106	+0.78
Lung Volumes: (Helium dilution)			
RV (L)	1.86	90	-0.58
FRC (L)	2.25	76	-1.40
TLC (L)	5.46	96	-0.38

All the SRs are between -1.64 and +1.64, so by scanning the SR column you can conclude "*Within normal limits*" after looking at the results for only a few seconds.

Patient 2.03 presented with breathlessness. There were basal crackles on auscultation of the lungs and a chest radiograph revealed diffuse lung shadowing.

PATIENT 2.03

Sex	Male	Height (m)	1.64
Age (yrs)	46	Weight (kg)	58
Tobacco	Ex-smoker	BMI (kg/m²)	22

	Measured	*% Predicted*	*SR*
Spirometry:			
FEV1 (L)	1.95	60	-2.51
VC (L)	2.20	56	-2.80
FEV1/VC (%)	89	112	+1.35

This clearly shows abnormal FEV1 and VC, with absolute SRs of more than 1.64.

The sign for both is negative, so both are low. The absolute SR for FEV1/VC is less than 1.64 and so this ratio is normal. As we will discuss further in the next chapter, low FEV and VC with a normal (or high) FEV1/VC indicates a restrictive defect. You could report these results as *"Restrictive defect"*. We could go futher and say *"Restrictive defect consistent with interstitial lung disease"*, taking account of the clinical information we are given. We might even make a few suggestions for further tests: *"Restrictive defect consistent with interstitial lung disease. Suggest measurement of full lung volumes, gas transfer and arterial blood gases."*

MILD, MODERATE OR SEVERE?

Having decided that a defect is present, how can we assess its severity? Compare Patient 2.04 with the previous example. Which patient has the more severe problem?

PATIENT 2.04

Sex	Female		Height (m)	1.45
Age (yrs)	37		Weight (kg)	39
Tobacco	Non-smoker		BMI (kg/m²)	19

	Measured	*% Predicted*	*SR*
Spirometry:			
FEV1 (L)	0.65	29	-4.08
VC (L)	0.65	25	-4.46
FEV1/VC (%)	100	123	+2.76

Here again FEV1 and VC are low, with a high FEV1/VC, but the absolute SRs are much greater. This indicates a greater deviation from normal, but how do we quantify this? *Mild*, *moderate* and *severe* are terms commonly used, but different ranges of percent predicted have been applied to different parameters of lung function. For example, the ATS definition of a severe defect is less than 50% of predicted for FVC but less than 40% of predicted for FEV1[4]. Most of the work on the severity of disability has been performed in airflow obstruction and has concentrated on FEV1.

One popular subdivision is as follows:

Severity:	*Percent predicted FEV1:*
Mild	60-79% predicted
Moderate	41-59% predicted
Severe	< 41% predicted

(Some alternatives have additional categories for "Moderately severe", "Very severe" and so on, but three subdivisions are usually sufficient.)

Percent predicted and SRs are not interchangeable, as we noted when looking at normal ranges. Unfortunately, use of SRs to assess the severity of disability has not yet been validated. Figure 2.8 shows the SRs for FEV1 in 100 patients attending our laboratory, 25 in each of the *mild, moderate* and *severe* categories as defined above and 25 with an FEV1 greater than 80% predicted (i.e. "Normal"):

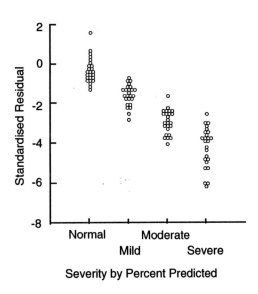

Figure 2.8

There is clearly a lot of overlap, but roughly equivalent grades we could use would be:

Severity:	*Standardised Residuals for FEV1:*
Mild	1.65 - 2.5
Moderate	2.51 - 3.50
Severe	>3.5

It seems reasonable to apply the same grades to VC (or TLC) when we are looking at a restrictive defect. With either SRs or % predicted, Patient 2.03 should then be reported as *"Moderately severe restrictive defect"* and Patient 2.04 as *"Severe restrictive defect"*.

A few final words about predicted values. I mentioned earlier the importance of using reference equations appropriate for the equipment used, ethnic group, etc.

Remember that at the extremes of age and height the number of individuals on whom the normal values are based may be very few. Try to get into the habit of scanning the patient's details at the top of the report, and look out for the very tall, the very short and the very old. Deviations from normality should then be interpreted with caution.

As the years go by, reference equations are progressively refined and expanded. The lungs of the population on which they are based can change subtly. Many of the early population studies included substantial numbers of individuals who smoked. In recent years, more data based exclusively on non-smokers has become available, and in the future this will probably become the basis of our reference equations. For the moment, interpretation of data from smokers involves a bit of guesswork to decide whether there is any damage from smoking or whether there is anything else going on. I shall touch on this question at various points in this book.

SUMMARY

☞ Standardised residuals (SRs) should be used to delineate normal from abnormal lung function tests.

☞ An absolute SR value >1.64 indicates that a test result is abnormal, negative values indicating an abnormally low test result and positive values an abnormally high result.

☞ If SRs are not available, <80% and >120% predicted can be used to identify abnormal lung function tests. However, some normal results will be classified as abnormal by these criteria.

☞ Severity of abnormality can be graded as follows:

	SR	*% Predicted*
Mild	1.65 - 2.5	60 - 79
Moderate	2.51 - 3.50	41 - 59
Severe	> 3.5	< 41

REFERENCES

1. Quanjer PhH. Standardised lung function testing - lung volumes and forced ventilatory flows. *Eur Respir J* 1993;**6**(suppl16):27.

2. Quanjer PhH. Standardised lung function testing - lung volumes and forced ventilatory flows. *Eur Respir J* 1993;**6**(suppl16):26.

3. Miller MR, Pincock AC. Predicted values: how should we use them? *Thorax* 1988;**43**:265–267.

4. American Thoracic Society. Evaluation of impairment/disability secondary to respiratory disorders. *Am Rev Respir Dis* 1992;**126**:945–951.

3: SPIROMETRY

Having ascertained how we define normality, we can now begin to recognise different patterns of abnormality. Even when other lung volumes and gas transfer data are available, the first step in analysis is to look at the simple spirometry.

AIRFLOW OBSTRUCTION

If the FEV1 is reduced and the ratio of FEV1 to VC is low, then airflow obstruction is present. (In this context, the VC used may be forced expiratory, relaxed expiratory or inspiratory, as we shall discuss later in this chapter.) A low FEV1/VC ratio is one that is below the lower limit of the normal range calculated for that individual, with an SR of less than -1.64; if the SR or normal range are not available, an FEV1 of less than 75% of VC is sometimes used to identify airflow obstruction, but this is a very rough rule of thumb which is particularly prone to error in the elderly, as we shall see shortly.

Bearing this in mind, and our definitions of severity from the previous chapter, how would you report the following spirometry results obtained in the pre-operative assessment of a patient awaiting cholecystectomy?

PATIENT 3.01

Sex:	Female	Height (m):	1.59
Age (yrs):	42	Weight (kg):	71
Tobacco:	Smoker	BMI (kg/m²):	28

	Measured	% Predicted	SR
Spirometry:			
FEV1 (L)	0.95	36	-4.42
VC (L)	2.15	70	-2.12
FEV1/VC (%)	44	54	-5.67

Both FEV1 and FEV1/VC ratio are low, so this is an obstructive defect. The absolute SR for FEV1 is more than 3.5 so our report should read *"Severe obstructive defect"*. The volume-time trace from this patient looks like this:

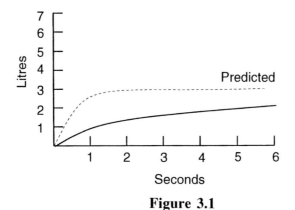

Figure 3.1

Note that the VC is also reduced, although not by as much as FEV1. This may be caused by collapse of airways during forced expiration, resulting in air trapping. VC may also be reduced if the test is terminated before the patient has finished exhaling, as we shall discuss at the end of this chapter when we look at the volume-time traces.

Sometimes a relaxed (expiratory) vital capacity (RVC) or even the inspiratory vital capacity (IVC) may also be given in the test results. Either of these may be considerably larger than the FVC in patients with airflow obstruction. FEV1/RVC or FEV1/IVC then give lower ratios than FEV1/FVC. (IVC is not easily measured on the traditional wedge bellows spirometer, making universal usage of FEV1/IVC difficult. This may change as the use of small computerized spirometers becomes more widespread.) Paradoxically, FVC may sometimes be greater than RVC, and in my view it is best to express FEV1 as a percentage of whichever is largest - IVC, FVC or RVC. This is what I mean by VC in all the spirometry examples in this book.

Patient 3.02 was admitted for repair of an abdominal aortic aneurysm. Do you think he has airflow obstruction?

PATIENT 3.02

Sex:	Male		Height (m):	1.68
Age (yrs):	75		Weight (kg):	64
Tobacco:	Smoker		BMI (kg/m²):	23

	Measured	*% Predicted*	*SR*
Spirometry:			
FEV1 (L)	2.15	84	-0.80
VC (L)	3.25	96	-0.23
FEV1/VC (%)	66	90	-1.05

Although FEV1/VC is only 66%, this is normal for a man of this age, as indicated by the SR. Our report must read *"Within normal limits"* - remember that the expected value of FEV1/VC declines with age (as a consequence of loss of lung elastic recoil force, as we shall see later), and should always be compared to the predicted value in the same way as other lung volumes:

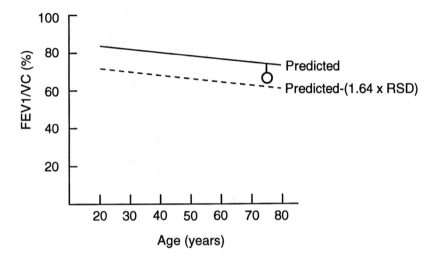

Figure 3.2

We saw in the previous chapter that many different parameters can be derived from simple spirometry data. Whilst some of these are of value in epidemiological surveys, for example to detect early airflow obstruction, most are of little value in clinical practice. The mean mid-expiratory flow (MMEF or FEF 25-75) has its advocates as a measure of small airways disease, but the normal range is very wide and interpretation of an abnormal result in the presence of a normal FEV1 must be made with caution. Individual labs may wish to incorporate this or another extra parameter in spirometry reports, but I shall not discuss them further here. The data can usually be retrieved easily from a modern computerised lung function test system if you think it would be useful to know in any individual case.

RESTRICTION

Patient 3.03 shows the other common pattern of spirometric abnormality, recorded in a patient with fibrosing alveolitis:

PATIENT 3.03

Sex:	Male	Height (m):	1.62
Age (yrs):	52	Weight (kg):	56
Tobacco:	Non-smoker	BMI (kg/m²):	21

	Measured	*% Predicted*	*SR*
Spirometry:			
FEV1 (L)	1.95	66	-2.00
VC (L)	2.20	60	-2.36
FEV1/VC (%)	89	114	+1.50

The volume-time trace looks like this:

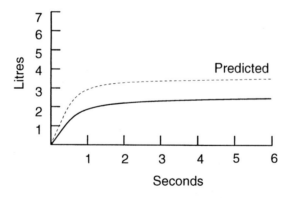

Figure 3.3

Both FEV1 and VC are reduced (SRs < -1.64), with a normal FEV1/VC ratio (again using SRs for the ratio, or an FEV1 > 75% of VC as a rough rule of thumb, to eliminate an obstructive component). This is the typical pattern of a restrictive defect, seen in many fibrotic lung diseases or when the lungs are compressed by an extra-pulmonary process, so we should report *"Restrictive defect"*. In a restrictive defect we look at VC to assess severity; bearing in mind our arbitrary definition of "Mild" as an SR of 1.65-2.5, we should report *"Mild restrictive defect"*.

If we define a restrictive defect as a low FEV1 and VC with a normal or high ratio, what do we do about patients with a low FEV1 but normal ratio?

PATIENT 3.04

Sex:	Female	Height (m):	1.66
Age (yrs):	52	Weight (kg):	68
Tobacco:	Non-smoker	BMI (kg/m²):	24

	Measured	*% Predicted*	*SR*
Spirometry:			
FEV (L)	1.96	73	-1.84
VC (L)	2.64	84	-1.11
FEV1/VC(%)	74	93	-0.76

Is this restriction, that is so mild that VC is not yet abnormal, or is it obstruction which is not severe enough to cause FEV1/VC to be low? The answer is that it is impossible to know what is going on, but whatever it is must be pretty mild. A reasonable report might be *"Slightly low FEV1. In presence of a normal VC and FEV1/VC ratio this is unlikely to be of any clinical significance, but if the patient is symptomatic it would probably be helpful to measure full lung volumes"*. As we shall see shortly, changes in RV and TLC should help to clarify this.

A similarly cautious interpretation should be made of a low VC with normal FEV1 and FEV1/VC ratio.

You may have noticed in Patient 3.03 that the ratio of FEV1 to VC was greater than predicted (SR > 0 and % Predicted > 100%), although still within the normal range (SR < +1.64). The elasticity of the lungs is an important factor in determining the maximum flow down an airway. For our present purposes, the exact mechanism is unimportant - the "equal pressure point" theory may be familiar from physiology textbooks, and the physics of viscoelastic flow are also involved. Patients with stiff lungs can produce airflow rates higher than normal, and the FEV1/VC may even have an SR > +1.64. (More of this in the chapters on peak expiratory flow rates and flow-volume loops).

ISOLATED ABNORMALITIES OF FEV1/VC

Sometimes FEV1/VC is abnormally low despite both FEV1 and VC themselves being within the normal range, as in this man who had a medical examination prior to employment as a diver:

PATIENT 3.05

		Height (m):	1.75
Sex:	Male	Height (m):	1.75
Age (yrs):	29	Weight (kg):	72
Tobacco:	Smoker	BMI (kg/m²):	24

	Measured	% Predicted	SR
Spirometry:			
FEV1 (L)	3.45	82	-1.45
VC (L)	5.20	104	+0.34
FEV1/VC (%)	66	81	-2.18

This may be an indication to the presence of airflow obstruction, which must nevertheless be very mild given the normal FEV1. In an asymptomatic subject, this is unlikely to be of any relevance[1], but might give a clue as to the aetiology of breathlessness on exercise, for example. A reasonable report might be *"Normal FEV1 and VC but slightly low FEV1/VC. This may indicate mild airflow obstruction, but should probably be ignored unless the subject is symptomatic"*. In a later chapter we shall see the value of looking at RV to confirm the suspicion of airflow obstruction in this context.

What if the ratio of FEV1 to VC is greater than normal, with an FEV1 and VC both within the normal range?

PATIENT 3.06

		Height (m):	1.55
Sex:	Female	Height (m):	1.55
Age (yrs):	54	Weight (kg):	62
Tobacco:	Non-smoker	BMI (kg/m²):	26

	Measured	% Predicted	SR
Spirometry:			
FEV1 (L)	2.55	117	+1.00
VC (L)	2.65	103	+0.19
FEV1/VC (%)	96	122	+2.67

Following on from the explanation of a high FEV1 to VC ratio in fibrosing alveolitis, you might suppose that these indicate early interstitial lung disease, at a stage when VC and FEV1 are still well preserved. In fact, this is almost never the case, and an isolated high FEV1/VC ratio should be ignored. *"Within normal limits"* is not strictly correct, since FEV1/VC is above the upper limit of normal, but *"No significant abnormality"* would be a reasonable report. A slightly fuller version could be *"Normal spirometry; high FEV1/VC ratio unlikely to be of any clinical significance"*. It would be worth checking on the volume-time trace that the manoeuvre was not terminated prematurely, giving a VC which is spuriously low for that individual, despite being within the normal range.

Whilst we are on the topic of supra-normal results, neither an abnormally high FEV1 nor VC point to any significant clinical abnormality, as in this highly-trained rower:

PATIENT 3.07

Sex:	Male	Height (m):	1.75
Age (yrs):	29	Weight (kg):	85
Tobacco:	Non-smoker	BMI (kg/m^2):	28

	Measured	*% Predicted*	*SR*
Spirometry:			
FEV1 (L)	6.50	155	+4.53
VC (L)	7.70	154	+4.44
FEV1/VC (%)	84	103	+0.34

MIXED OBSTRUCTIVE/RESTRICTIVE DEFECTS

When we discussed airflow obstruction earlier in this chapter, we observed that VC is often low in this pattern of defect. Sometimes you will see this reported as a mixed obstructive/restrictive problem. Clearly some patients will have both types of problem, for example in a smoker who develops fibrosing alveolitis, but it is very difficult to infer this from spirometry alone. We shall return to this problem in the chapter on lung volumes.

REVERSIBILITY

If spirometry shows an obstructive defect, the measurements will often be repeated after administration of an inhaled bronchodilator to see if the defect is reversible. (Some units routinely measure spirometry before and after bronchodilators even if the initial results are normal, on the grounds that the normal range is sufficiently wide that an individual may be well below their best and yet still within the normal range).

Do you think that the change in Patient 3.08's FEV1 implies that his airflow obstruction is reversible or not?

PATIENT 3.08

Sex:	Male	Height (m):	1.63
Age (yrs):	69	Weight (kg):	78
Tobacco:	Smoker	BMI (kg/m²):	29

	Measured	*After Salbutamol*
Spirometry:		
FEV1 (L)	0.70	0.85

There is some controversy about how best to detect significant reversibility. Obviously the amount of change must be greater than the variability of the test. For FEV1 this is about 0.20 L[2]. We should therefore report *"No significant improvement in FEV1 after salbutamol"*.

There has been considerable debate about other methods of expressing changes in FEV1 after bronchodilators[3]. Probably the most common method is to express the increase after bronchodilators as a percentage of the baseline value, with 15% as the cut-off above which reversibility is taken to be significant. With this system, only a small change in FEV1 is required of a patient with very severe airflow obstruction to say they are reversible, and this change may even be less than the reproducibility of the test. In our example, the increase of 0.15 L is 21% of the pre-bronchodilator value:

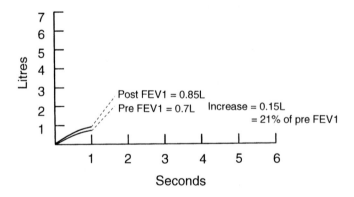

Figure 3.4

A patient with a larger FEV1 may show a considerable improvement after bronchodilators which is nevertheless less than 15%:

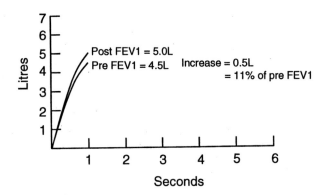

Figure 3.5

In order to overcome this problem, the European Respiratory Society (ERS) recommend expressing any increase in FEV1 as a percentage of the predicted value, using >12% as the cut-off for significant reversibility[4]. This alternative is becoming increasingly widely used.

Always bear in mind that if the short-term bronchodilator assessment in the lung function laboratory has not shown any significant change, this does not necessarily mean that the airflow obstruction is irreversible. A longer trial of treatment at home may have beneficial effects, and it would be wrong to label the patient "irreversible" in our report. *"No significant reversibility demonstrated"* is a better phrase to use.

Reversibility is sometimes defined by an increase in VC (FVC or RVC), with or without an increase in FEV1. Let us look at what happened to VC in our patient:

PATIENT 3.08

Sex:	Male	Height (m):	1.63
Age (yrs):	69	Weight (kg):	78
Tobacco:	Smoker	BMI (kg/m²):	29

	Measured	*After Salbutamol*
Spirometry:		
FEV1 (L)	0.7	0.85
VC (L)	2.1	2.35
FEV1/VC (%)	33	36

We have already noted the problems of measuring VC in patients with airflow obstruction, and any clinically significant reversibility is likely to reflected by an increase in FEV1. There seems little point in confusing matters by adding in VC, but if you are going to take it into consideration, the increase must be greater than the reproducibility of the test. In expert hands, repeated measurements of VC can be within 0.2 L, but an increase of 0.35 L is often used as the cut-off. In our patient, the increase in VC is less than this, so our conclusion should remain unchanged.

Let us suppose that VC had increased, with little change in FEV1:

PATIENT 3.08

Sex:	Male	Height (m):	1.63
Age (yrs):	69	Weight (kg):	78
Tobacco:	Smoker	BMI (kg/m²):	29

	Measured	*After Salbutamol*
Spirometry:		
FEV1 (L)	0.7	0.85
VC (L)	2.1	2.9
FEV1/VC (%)	33	29

Note that the ratio of FEV1 to VC actually falls. Although the ratio of FEV1 to VC is the main index we look at to determine the presence of airflow obstruction, it should not be used to assess whether or not there is any reversibility.

SGaw (see Chapter 6) and mid-expiratory flow rates can also be used to assess reversibility, but their reproducibility is such that again they add little to FEV1.

BRONCHIAL REACTIVITY

We have looked at how to assess increases in airway calibre after inhalation of bronchodilators. The other side of the coin is how airways react to a bronchoconstrictor. Cold air, exercise, or an allergen can be used, but the most common stimulus is inhalation of a drug such as methacholine or histamine[5]. After recording a baseline FEV1, increasing amounts of the bronchoconstrictor agent are inhaled by the subject until the FEV1 has fallen by 20% of the initial value. If this happens with a very small amount of methacholine or histamine, the airways are "hyperreactive" and the patient probably has asthma.

There are two main ways of administering these bronchoconstrictor agents. Dosimeters, either electronic or hand held, administer a small dose of the agent to the subject at the start of a breath in[6]. The size of each dose is known, so a record can be kept of the total cumulative dose inhaled. The amount which produces a fall in FEV1 of 20% is then known as the Provocative Dose or PD_{20}. The alternative method uses a conventional nebuliser[7]. The subject breathes tidally from the nebulizer for a fixed period of time, then records an FEV1 and if there has not been a fall of 20% then they move on immediately to a higher concentration. The effects of each period of nebulisation are cumulative, but it is difficult to calculate exactly how much of the agent has been inhaled by the subject. With this method the reactivity of the airways is therefore better expressed as the Provocative Concentration which produced a 20% fall in FEV1, or PC_{20}.

Patient 3.09 had a chronic cough for which no cause was apparent after clinical examination, a chest radiograph and spirometry. A histamine challenge test was performed using the nebulisation method:

PATIENT 3.09

		FEV1 (L)
Baseline		2.89
Diluent		2.82
Histamine	0.03	2.91
(mg/ml)	0.06	2.96
	0.13	2.88
	0.25	2.83
	0.50	2.79
	1.00	2.21

We can plot these results and by interpolation derive the concentration of histamine which caused a 20% fall in FEV1:

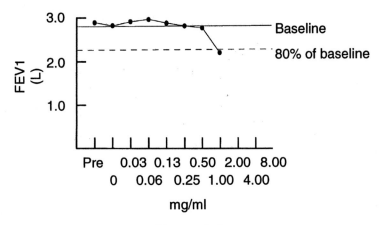

Figure 3.6

In a normal subject, the PC_{20} should be at least 8mg/ml. (For the dosimeter method a normal PD_{20} is >4 micromoles.) In our patient bronchoconstriction occurs at a much lower concentration of histamine, so their airways are hyperreactive. In this clinical context, we suspect that the cough is caused by asthma.

VOLUME-TIME TRACE ABNORMALITIES

If patient 3.01 stopped expiring after 1.5 seconds, we would have erroneously found a restrictive defect, with the ratio of FEV1 to VC being high:

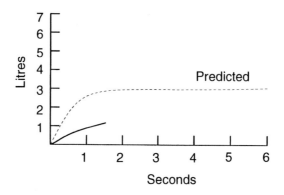

Figure 3.7

Obviously we would have spotted this error in technique when he performed the test, but subtler variants of this problem may be seen with computerised spirometers which terminate the test after a few seconds, irrespective of whether expiration is complete. This can often be spotted by looking at the volume-time trace, where it will be seen that the trace is still sloping upwards at the end of the test. Whenever possible you should look at the volume-time trace, to see how well the patient has performed the test, and note any comments made on the trace by the technicians. A technical problem with the spirometer, poor patient technique or poor effort are often easily apparent (figure 3.8).

A comment such as *"Poor patient technique - volumes likely to be underestimated"* at some stage in our report would be appropriate.

Figure 3.9 shows a linear trace, with little change in slope during the manoeuvre. The slope of the trace is change in volume with time, i.e. flow, which in this case is independant of lung volume. This points to large airway obstruction and is an indication to perform a flow-volume loop (see Chapter 5).

A similar pattern may be seen in severe emphysema. The difference in Figure 3.10 is that there is a short curvilinear portion at the onset of expiration, corresponding to the initial peak in flow which is characteristic of this condition on a flow-volume loop:

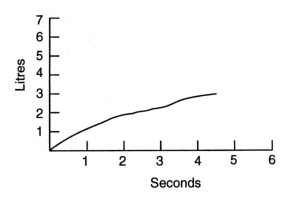

Figure 3.8

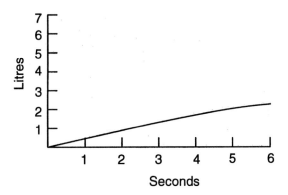

Figure 3.9

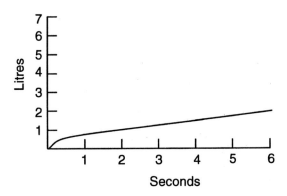

Figure 3.10

Figure 3.11 shows a rarer trace, with two distict phases. One part of the lungs is emptying much more slowly than the remainder. This pattern is seen very occasionally in patients with a single lung transplant for emphysema, or with stenosis of a main bronchus[8].

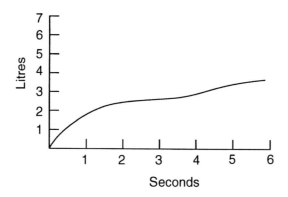

Figure 3.11

SUMMARY

☞ An obstructive defect is characterized by a low FEV1 and low FEV1 to VC ratio. VC may also be low.

☞ The normal ratio of FEV1 to VC declines with age, and FEV1/VC should be compared to the predicted value in the same way as any other lung function test.

☞ A restrictive defect consists of a low FEV1 and VC with a normal or high ratio of FEV1 to VC.

☞ If the FEV1 and VC are within the normal range, an abnormal FEV1/VC ratio should be ignored.

☞ Reversibility to bronchodilators is best defined as an increase in FEV1 of more than 0.2L. A additional requirement for the increase to be more than 12% of the predicted FEV1 is increasingly comonly used.

☞ Failure to demonstrate reversibility in the lung function laboratory over a few minutes does not necessarily mean that the airflow obstruction is never reversible.

☞ Bronchial hyperreactivity is present if the PC_{20} for histamine or methacholine is less than 8 mg/ml using the nebulizer method, or the PD_{20} is less than 4 micromoles for the dosimeter method.

REFERENCES

1. Kivity S, Solomon A, Schwarz Y, Trajber I, Topilsky M. Evaluation of asymptomatic subjects with low forced expiratory ratios (FEV1/VC). *Thorax* 1994;**49**:554–556.

2. Tweedale PM, Alexander F, McHardy GJR. Short term variability in FEV1 and bronchodilator responsiveness in patients with obstructive ventilatory defects. *Thorax* 1987;**42**:487–490.

3. Dompeling E, van Schayck CP, Molema J, Akkermans R, Folgering H, van Grunsven PM, van Weel C. A comparison of six different ways of expressing the bronchodilating response in asthma and COPD; reproducibility and dependence of prebronchodilator FEV1. *Eur Respir J* 1992;**5**:975–981.

4. Quanjer PhH. Standardised lung function testing - lung volumes and forced ventilatory flows. *Eur Respir J* 1993;**6**(suppl16):p24.

5. Sterk PJ, Fabbri LM. Quanjer PhH, Cockcroft DW, O'Byrne PM, Anderson SD, Juniper EF, Malo J-F. Airway responsiveness. *Eur Respir J* 1993;6 Suppl **16**:53–83.

6. Yan K, Salomw C, Woolcock AJ. Rapid method for measurement of bronchial responsiveness. *Thorax* 1983;**38**:760–765.

7. Cockcroft DW, Killian DN, Mellon JJA, Hargreave FE. Bronchial reactivity to inhaled histamine: a method and clinical survey. *Clin Allergy* 1977;**7**:235–243.

8. Gascoigne AD, Corris PA, Dark JH, Gibson GJ. The biphasic spirogram: a clue to unilateral narrowing of a mainstem bronchus. *Thorax* 1990;**45**:637–638.

4: PEAK EXPIRATORY FLOW RATES

Serial measurements of PEFR are central to the management of asthma, both for diagnosis and monitoring the response to treatment[1,2]. You may have noticed that I did not give PEFR data along with FEV1 and VC in the previous chapter, and possibly be puzzled as to why we are considering this simple test after spirometry. My reason for doing this is that a single PEFR recording is seldom useful in diagnosis, particularly if other lung function data are available, and in order to justify this viewpoint we needed to fully undertand spirometry first.

On the basis of their PEFR, which of Patients 4.01 to 4.04 would you say has airflow obstruction?

	Measured	*% Predicted*	*SR*
Patient 4.01			
PEFR (L/min)	255	50	-3.50
Patient 4.02			
PEFR (L/min)	200	56	-2.90
Patient 4.03			
PEFR (L/min)	330	72	-2.30
Patient 4.04			
PEFR (L/min)	290	61	-2.50

Clearly all have low PEFRs, with SRs of less than -1.64, and on the basis of this alone all could be said to have airflow obstruction.

However, look at the data again along with their spirometry:

	Measured	% Predicted	SR
Patient 4.01			
FEV1 (L)	1.55	46	-3.62
VC (L)	2.89	67	-2.31
FEV/VC (%)	54	70	-3.23
PEFR (L/min)	255	50	-3.50
Patient 4.02			
FEV1 (L)	1.00	42	-3.50
VC (L)	1.23	44	-3.55
FEV1/VC (%)	81	103	+0.46
PEFR (L/min)	200	56	-2.90
Patient 4.03			
FEV1 (L)	1.60	45	-5.08
VC (L)	1.75	43	-5.35
FEV1/VC (%)	91	109	+1.18
PEFR (L/min)	330	72	-2.30
Patient 4.04			
FEV1 (L)	1.72	57	-2.53
VC (L)	2.20	58	-2.57
FEV1/VC (%)	78	102	+0.20
PEFR (L/min)	290	61	-2.50

Patient 4.01 does indeed have airflow obstruction, confirmed by the low FEV1/VC ratio, whereas Patient 4.02 has restriction secondary to pulmonary fibrosis. Although the latter's PEFR is low, FEV1/VC is within normal limits, showing that there is no airflow obstruction but that the low PEFR is simply a reflection of the low lung volume at which the manoeuvre was performed. Similarly, patient 4.03 has a severe thoracic scoliosis and Patient 4.04 has a paralysed hemi-diaphragm - neither has airflow obstruction.

You can demonstrate the effect of lung volume on expiratory flow easily with a peak flow meter yourself. Inspire to TLC and then blow hard and note your peak flow ("A" in Figure 4.1). Then take a much smaller breath, say to about half a litre above FRC, then blow hard into the peak flow meter again ("B"). Your peak flow will be much lower on the second occassion.

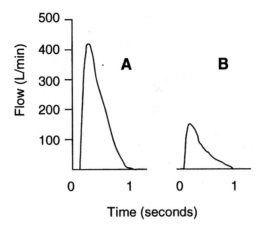

Figure 4.1

We noted in the first part of this chapter that patients with restrictive defects can have an FEV1/VC ratio greater than normal. If we superimpose Patient 4.03's PEFR manoeuvre (——) on the predicted expiratory flow-volume curve (- - - -) (figure 4.2), you will see that her PEFR is actually greater than would be expected at that lung volume (arrowed), even though it is well below the normal range for the value which would be expected if she could inspire to a normal TLC:

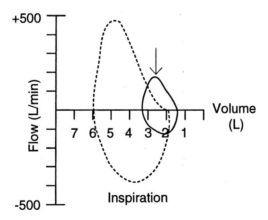

Figure 4.2

Thus the PEFR is difficult to interpret if the VC is low. The unwary may erroneously interpret a low PEFR as indicating airflow obstruction in a patient with restrictive lung disease (or in neuromuscular disease, as we will see in the chapter on flow-volume loops) and in my view it would probably be better if this measurement were to be omitted from lung function test results.

REVERSIBILITY

In the chapter on spirometry, we discussed testing reversibility to inhaled bronchodilators. Peak flow can also be used to assess reversibility, although it is usually measured together with spirometry. As with FEV1, to be significant any increase must be greater than the spontaneous variability of repeated measurements made in the same subject on the same day. In this context, an increase in PEFR of 60 L/min or more can be used to detect reversible airflow obstruction[3,4]. The same debate arises as for FEV1 about expressing the change as percent of the initial value, percent predicted, etc. It is probably best to give the change in L/min and leave it to the clinician involved to decide whether or not the change represents any useful clinical benefit, taking into account the patient's overall function.

SUMMARY

☞ A low PEFR is an unreliable way of detecting airflow obstruction.

☞ An increase in PEFR of >60L/min after bronchodilator can be used to define significant reversibility.

REFERENCES

1. Lebowitz MP, Quanjer PhH. Peak expiratory flow. *Eur Respir J* 1997;**10**(suppl 24):1s–83s.

2. Ayres JG, Turpin PJ. *Peak flow measurement*. Chapman and Hall, London 1997.

3. Dekker FW, Schrier AC, Sterk PJ, Dijkman JH. Validity of peak flow measurement in assessing reversibility of airflow obstruction. *Thorax* 1992;**47**:162–166.

4. Hegewald MJ, Crapo RO, Jensen RL. Intraindividual peak flow variability. *Chest* 1995;**107**:156–161.

5: FLOW-VOLUME LOOPS

In Chapter 3 we saw that the pattern of a spirogram may suggest that airflow obstruction is the result of a lesion in the upper rather than lower airways. The best test to perform next would be a flow volume loop, and indeed this should always be requested if there is a suspicion of upper airway obstruction. For some reason, many people regard flow-volume loops as incomprehensible, and they generate a great deal of anxiety in the minds of exam candidates. If you understand how the manoeuvre is performed, all that is required is to become familiar with a fairly small number of shapes which the curve can take. Disorientation is less of a problem for the unfamiliar if "Inspiration", "Expiration", "TLC" and "RV" are all clearly marked on the trace, but this is not always the case. One other source of confusion is that the flow scale is usually given in litres per second, whereas on the wards we are much more familiar with peak flows recorded in litres per minute.

THE FLOW-VOLUME MANOEUVRE

When a flow-volume loop is recorded, the patient is asked to breathe in to TLC. They then perform a forced expiration down to RV, then breathe in back to TLC again. In papers and books, the noise on these traces is usually filtered out, so don't be surprised if the flow-volume loops you report on are much more "jagged" in appearance.

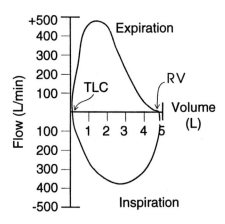

Figure 5.1

If RV is known, from either helium dilution or plethysmography (see next chapter), the loop can be plotted with absolute lung volume on the X-axis:

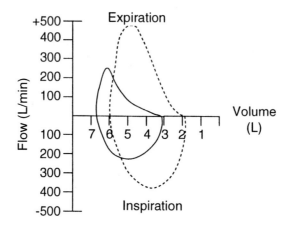

Figure 5.2

Comparison with the predicted loop shows how TLC, RV and VC (TLC minus RV) are affected by the disease process, in this case airflow obstruction, together with the expiratory and inspiratory flow patterns. Not many computerised lung function testing systems support this presentation of flow-volume loops, which is a shame, given the amount of information that it contains. (A further refinement has two horizontal bars for transfer factor and alveolar volume[1]).

AIRWAY OBSTRUCTION

On the trace in Figure 5.1, notice that the latter part of the expiratory loop has a smooth concave shape. Over this region of the loop, flow is limited by airway calibre rather than patient effort. In patients with airflow obstruction in the "lower" or intra-thoracic airways, the concave part of the curve begins much sooner in expiration, as we have just seen:

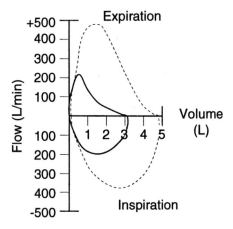

Figure 5.3

Patients with "laryngeal" wheeze, who start to wheeze when someone in a white coat approaches the end of their bed, have very variable and irregular flow-volume loops, which are usually easy to distinguish from a true asthmatic pattern[2,3].

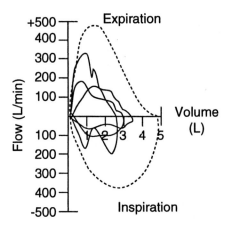

Figure 5.4

When this type of obstruction to flow in the lower airways is more severe, for example in emphysema, the concave part of the expiratory curve begins very early in expiration:

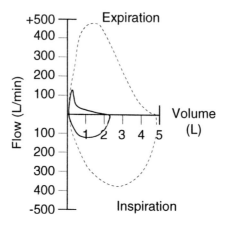

Figure 5.5

Notice in this patient that during inspiration, flow is more like the normal pattern. The negative intra-thoracic pressure during inspiration holds the floppy airways open, and there is a marked difference between inspiratory and expiratory flows.

FIXED LARGE AIRWAY OBSTRUCTION

Contrast Figure 5.5 with what happens when the trachea is concentrically narrowed by a tumour:

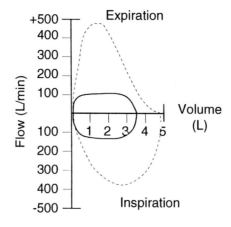

Figure 5.6

Here the narrow tracheal segment is rigid, with no compression during expiration and no dilation during inspiration. As a result, inspiratory and expiratory flows are much more similar. The expiratory curve does not have the concave shape that we noted previously: the degree of airflow obstruction does not vary with intra-thoracic pressure and lung volume, so a flat expiratory plateau is seen. Inspiratory flow is also flat, giving a characteristic box-like shape to the flow-volume loop. This pattern is seen with any rigid concentric lesion anywhere between the carina and the mouth[4,5].

VARIABLE LARGE AIRWAY OBSTRUCTION

If a less rigid lesion obstructs a major airway, the pattern of flow-volume loop varies with the site of the obstruction. If the obstruction is "intrathoracic", i.e. below the supra-sternal notch, the degree of obstruction will tend to be exacerbated during expiration when intra-thoracic pressure is positive and alleviated during inspiration when negative intrathoracic pressure dilates the obstructing lesion.

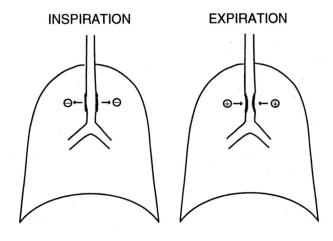

Figure 5.7

The same plateaus will be seen as in a rigid concentric lesion, particularly during expiration:

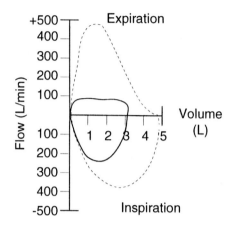

Figure 5.8

A similar lesion which is "extra-thoracic", i.e. above the supra-sternal notch, will show the opposite tendency. Since it is outside the thorax, it will not be influenced by intra-thoracic pressure[6]. However, the positive intra-luminal pressure during expiration will tend to dilate the lesion and alleviate the obstruction.

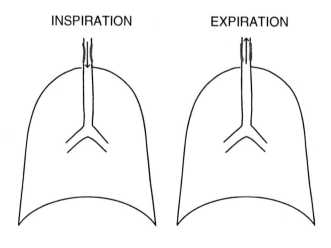

Figure 5.9

During inspiration, the Bernouille effect will tend to collapse the lesion and exacerbate the obstruction. Flow is generally independant of lung volume, so plateaus are seen, in this case with expiratory flow being greater than inspiratory flow:

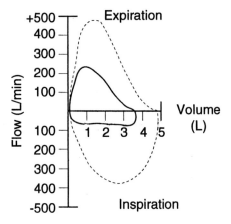

Figure 5.10

Very occasionally, a lesion at the level of the supra-sternal notch will behave like an extra-thoracic lesion at TLC but by RV be intra-thoracic[4]. The transition from one compartment to the other during expiration gives a characterisitic notch on the flow-volume loop:

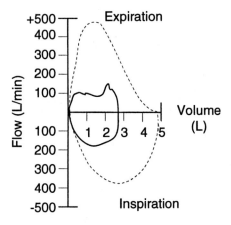

Figure 5.11

Performing a maximal inspiration immediately after forced expiration can be quite difficult, and on many of the loops you see the starting volume is not reached:

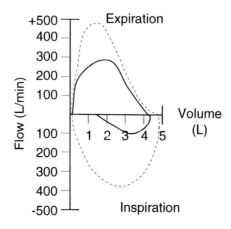

Figure 5.12

The only relevance of this is that a slightly flat inspiratory loop should be interpreted with some caution if the inspiratory volume is much less than the expiratory volume.

NEUROMUSCULAR DISEASE

Inspiratory flow limitation can also be seen in patients with "floppiness" of the vocal cords or pharynx[7]. Complete phayrngeal collapse may cause notching of the inspiratory limb[8]:

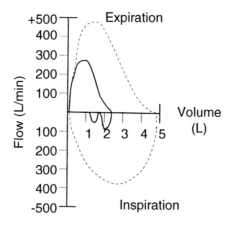

Figure 5.13

Notching on both inspiratory and expiratory limbs can be seen in patients with dystonic muscular activity[9]:

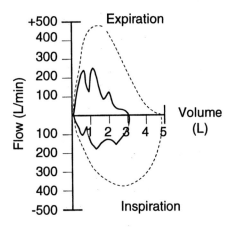

Figure 5.14

The concavity of a normal expiratory flow-volume loop shows that flow is independant of patient effort: blowing harder doesn't produce more flow, because the airways only collapse more. During the early part of expiration, before the concave part of the curve is reached, flow is effort dependant. Weakness of the expiratory muscles may lead to blunting of the peak on the curve, which otherwise has a fairly normal shape, although there may also be a slight step as flow ceases fairly abruptly near RV[10]:

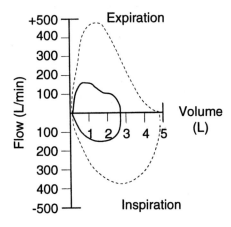

Figure 5.15

PHARYNGEAL FLUTTER

Inspiratory or expiratory flutter, manifest as saw-tooth oscillations on one or both limbs of the flow-volume trace, can also be seen in patients with bulbar weakness, and has also been reported in patients with a narrow pharynx who are prone to obstructive sleep apnoea[11]:

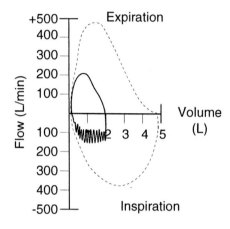

Figure 5.16

FIBROTIC LUNG DISEASE

We saw that in a normal subject, airway collapse gives a characteristic concave shape to the flow volume loop during the latter part of expiration. We also noted that in patients with narrow or more collapsable airways the point at which the expiratory curve becomes concave is reached much earlier in expiration. On the other hand, patients with fibrotic lung disease have airways which are less collapsable and the flow-volume loop only becomes concave right at the end of expiration:

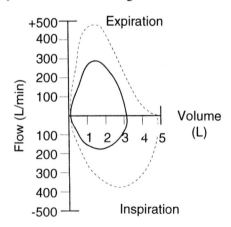

Figure 5.17

SOME RARER ABNORMALITIES

A two-phase flow-volume loop, where one lung, or part of a lung, empties more slowly. This can be seen with a stenosed bronchus, or when a patient with emphysema has had a single lung transplant[12]:

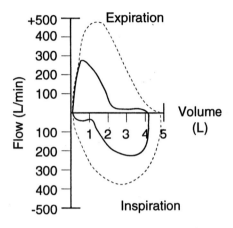

Figure 5.18

Transplantation causes an increase in expiratory flow, presumably because of denervation of the lung, with loss of tonic vagal vasoconstriction[13]:

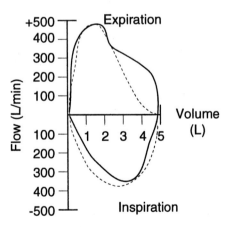

Figure 5.19

Obliterative bronchiolits has been documented to erase this pattern.

Tracheobronchomegaly has a characteristic flow-volume loop appearance, with the same general expiratory shape as an asthmatic, but with notches superimposed[5,14]:

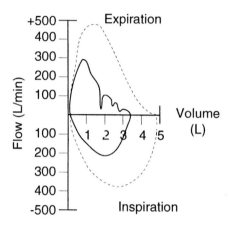

Figure 5.20

NUMERICAL INDICES

You may have noticed that I have only talked about the shape of the curves, not absolute values of flow, ratios of flow, etc. Many such parameters can be measured or calculated, but their utility is limited. They cannot reliably differentiate upper from lower airway obstruction[15], and it is much more important to look at the actual trace.

SUMMARY

☞   In generalized airflow obstruction, the expiratory limb of the FV loop is concave.

☞   In fibrotic lung disease or patients with expiratory muscle weakness, the expiratory limb of the FV loop is convex.

☞   Constricting lesions of the trachea and upper airway lead to box-shaped FV loops. If the lesion is complaint, expiratory flow will be greater than inspiratory if it is above the supra-sternal notch, vice-versa if below.

☞   Upper airway problems lead to coarse irregularities on the FV loop.

REFERENCES

1.   Denison DM, DuBois R, Sawicka E. Does the lung work ? Pictures in the mind. *Br J Dis Chest* 1983;**77**:35–50.

2.   Mobeirek A, Alhamad A, Al-Subaei A, Alzeer A. Psychogenic vocal cord dysfunction simulating bronchial asthma. *Eur Respir J* 1995;**8**:1978–1981.

3.   McFadden ER, Zawadski DK. Vocal cord dysfunction masquerading as exercise-induced asthma. *Am J Respir Crit Care Med* 1996;**153**:942–947.

4.   Harrison BWD. Upper airway obstruction - a report on sixteen patients. *Q J Med* 1976;**180**:625–645.

5.   Kryger M, Bode F, Antic R, Anthonisen N. Diagnosis of obstruction of the upper and central airways. *Am J Med* 1976;**61**:85–93.

6. Miller MR, Pincock AC, Oates GD, Wilkinson R, Skene-Smith H. Upper airway obstruction due to goitre: detection, prevalence and results of surgical management. *Q J Med* 1990;**74**:177–188.

7. Putman MT, Wise RA. Myasthenia gravis and upper airway obstruction. *Chest* 1996;**109**:400–404.

8. Garcia-Pachon E, Marti J, Mayos M, Casan P, Sanchis J. Clinical significance of upper airway dysfunction in motor neurone disease. *Thorax* 1994;**49**:896–900.

9. Braun N, Antoine A, Baer J, Blitzer A, Stewart C, Brin M. Dyspnoea in dystonia - a functional evaluation. *Chest* 1995;**107**:1309–1316.

10. Vincken W, Elleker G, Cosio MG. Detection of upper airway muscle involvement in neuromuscular disorders using the flow-volume loop. *Chest* 1986;**90**:52–57.

11. Sanders MH, Martin RJ, Pennock BE, Rogers RM. The detection of sleep apnoea in the awake patient. *JAMA* 1981;**245**:2414–2418.

12. Gascoigne AD, Corris PA, Dark JH, Gibson GJ. The biphasic spirogram: a clue to unilateral narrowing of a mainstem bronchus. *Thorax* 1990;**45**:637–638.

13. Estenne M, Ketelblant P, Primo G, Yernault J-C. Human heart-lung transplantation: physiologic aspects of the denervated lung and post-transplant obliterative bronchiolitis. *Am Rev Respir Dis* 1987;**135**:976–978.

14. Bonnet R, Jorres R, Downey R, Hein H, Magnussen H. Intractable cough associated with the supine body position. *Chest* 1995;**108**:581–585.

15. Rotman HH, Liss HP, Weg JG. Diagnosis of upper airway obstruction by pulmonary function testing. *Chest* 1975;**68**:796–799.

6: LUNG VOLUMES

Whilst spirometry gives us some idea about airflow and the size of the lungs, lung volumes (RV, FRC and TLC) give us a more detailed picture and may point to the underlying pathological disease process. These additional lung volumes are usually obtained either by helium dilution or plethysmography. For the moment, let's stick to the helium method.

HELIUM DILUTION

FRC is estimated by watching how the concentration of Helium falls when inspired gas with a known concentration of Helium is diluted as it equilibrates with the gas in the lungs:

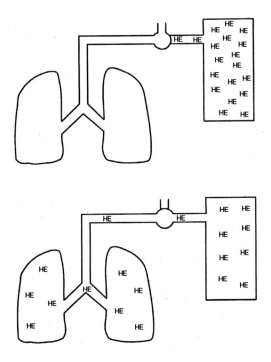

Figure 6.1

The inspired gas only equilibrates with the ventilated lung, so unventilated or very poorly ventilated parts of the lung will be missed.

RESTRICTION

By far the most common situation is for the lung volumes to confirm our initial impression formed on the basis of the spirometry results, as in this patient with breathlessness and diffuse lung shadowing on her chest radiograph:

PATIENT 6.01

Sex:	Female	Height (m):	1.73	
Age (yrs):	28	Weight (kg):	57	
Tobacco:	Non-smoker	BMI (kg/m^2):	19	

	Measured	% Predicted	SR
Spirometry:			
FEV1 (L)	1.60	45	-5.09
VC (L)	1.75	52	-5.34
FEV1/VC (%)	91	117	+1.17
Lung Volumes: (Helium dilution)			
RV (L)	0.87	42	-2.03
FRC (L)	1.30	44	-3.21
TLC (L)	2.62	46	-6.02

VC is reduced, with a normal FEV1 to VC ratio, typical of restriction. A restrictive defect can also be defined as a low TLC, so lung volumes confirm our initial impression. (TLC should take precedence over VC in deciding whether a restrictive defect is present, and in assessing severity.) In this case we should report *" Severe restrictive defect"* on the basis of the SR for TLC. Knowledge of lung volumes has not changed our interpretation of the defect seen on spirometry, although the very low TLC is reassuring evidence that this is indeed a severe restrictive defect.

The next patient was breathless on walking but spirometry showed only a mild abnormality. Lung volumes were therefore requested:

PATIENT 6.02

		Height (m):	1.45
Sex:	Female	Height (m):	1.45
Age (yrs):	62	Weight (kg):	67
Tobacco:	Non-smoker	BMI (kg/m²):	32

	Measured	% Predicted	SR
Spirometry:			
FEV1 (L)	0.99	63	-1.55
VC (L)	1.16	60	-1.77
FEV1/VC (%)	85	110	+1.23
Lung Volumes: (Helium dilution)			
RV (L)	0.67	41	-2.71
FRC (L)	1.03	45	-2.56
TLC (L)	1.79	47	-3.32

Here we might have been tempted to ignore the slightly low FVC, but full lung volumes clearly show that there is indeed a restrictive defect.

One step further takes us to the patient with normal spirometry in whom we continue to suspect that there is something wrong with their lungs:

PATIENT 6.03

Sex	Female	Height (m)	1.53
Age (yrs)	58	Weight (kg)	87
Tobacco	Non-smoker	BMI (kg/m²)	37

	Measured	% Predicted	SR
Spirometry:			
FEV1 (L)	2.20	111	+1.99
VC (L)	2.60	109	+0.51
FEV1/VC (%)	85	109	+1.00
Lung Volumes: (Helium dilution)			
RV (L)	0.96	56	-2.11
FRC (L)	1.12	45	-2.73
TLC (L)	3.56	83	-1.50

Spirometry is essentially normal, although we might note in passing that the FEV1 is slightly greater than normal. TLC is normal, but both FRC and RV are low. Is this a restrictive defect? A low RV (usually accompanied by a low FRC aswell) can be a pointer to parenchymal or pleural restriction[1]. The high FEV1 would support this interpretation, even though FEV1/VC is within the normal range. We might report these tests as *"No clear evidence of a restrictive or obstructive defect, but reduced RV and FRC can indicate an early pulmonary or pleural restrictive process. Measurement of gas transfer might be helpful"*.

OBSTRUCTION

The following results were obtained on a patient in whom the spirometry showed an obstructive defect:

PATIENT 6.04

Sex:	Male	Height (m):	1.82
Age (yrs):	49	Weight (kg):	88
Tobacco:	Smoker	BMI (kg/m^2):	24

	Measured	*% Predicted*	*SR*
Spirometry:			
FEV1 (L)	2.05	52	-3.66
VC (L)	4.25	87	-1.02
FEV1/VC (%)	48	61	-4.21
Lung Volumes: (Helium dilution)			
RV (L)	5.27	236	+7.41
FRC (L)	6.85	187	+5.40
TLC (L)	9.52	128	+3.43

There are a number of physiological reasons why the lung volumes are so high, the main ones being loss of inward elastic recoil force (as a result of emphysema) and air trapping. However changes in the compliance of the chest wall and respiratory muscles may also contribute. It is tempting to talk about "hyperinflation" in our report on a set of results such as these, but this means different things to different people. It can be used to signify an increase in FRC or in TLC. Moreover, it is difficult to aportion blame to the various pathophysiological processes without a lot more information, particularly about pleural pressure. Similar arguments apply to the term "air trapping", which is somtimes used when RV is high but TLC is less elevated.

It is probably safer therefore to stick to *"Severe airflow obstruction"* without making guesses about the balance between airway closure and loss of elastic recoil. In the next chapter we'll see how carbon monoxide transfer can lead us towards a diagnosis of asthma, emphysema or chronic bronchitis.

How do full lung volumes affect your interpretation of spirometry in the next patient?

PATIENT 6.05

Sex:	Male	Height (m):	1.62
Age (yrs):	50	Weight (kg):	72
Tobacco:	Smoker	BMI (kg/m²):	27

	Measured	*% Predicted*	*SR*
Spirometry:			
FEV1 (L)	2.35	78	-1.33
VC (L)	3.55	96	-0.23
FEV1/VC (%)	66	85	-1.68
Lung Volumes: (Helium dilution)			
RV (L)	3.11	156	+2.73
FRC (L)	3.81	121	+1.10
TLC (L)	6.66	114	+1.33

FEV1 and VC are both normal, although the FEV1/VC is slightly low, suggesting airflow obstruction. In a breathless smoker, we might wonder whether this is sufficient to explain his symptoms. However, when we look at the full lung volumes, our initial impression of airflow obstruction is considerably re-inforced by the finding of quite marked elevation of RV. We could report *"Low FEV1/VC and elevated RV suggest mild airflow obstruction"*. In this patient, additional lung volumes have given us more confidence in the impression we gained from spirometry.

When an elevated RV is the only abnormality, the most common explanation is early emphysema[2], although myopathies, chest wall deformity and heart failure must all be borne in mind. (We'll discuss some of these further when looking at RV/TLC).

PATIENT 6.06

Sex:	Male	Height (m):	1.79
Age (yrs):	58	Weight (kg):	86
Tobacco:	Smoker	BMI (kg/m²):	27

Clinical details: Breathless - cause?

	Measured	*% Predicted*	*SR*
Spirometry:			
FEV1 (L)	3.15	89	-0.75
VC (L)	4.35	97	-0.18
FEV1/VC (%)	72	94	-0.61
Lung Volumes: (Helium dilution)			
RV (L)	3.33	139	+2.29
FRC (L)	3.80	105	+0.30
TLC (L)	7.68	106	+0.66

A cautious interpretation might be *"Elevated RV suggests mild emphysema or airflow obstruction. Other alternative explanations to consider are thoracic deformity, expiratory muscle weakness and heart failure".*

PLETHYSMOGRAPHY

Let's now look at the other method commonly used to measure lung volumes. In a constant volume body plethysmograph, the volume of gas in the thorax is estimated by the swings in pressure in the box (pressure guage A: figure 6.2) when the subject compresses the gas slightly (as indicated by pressure gauge B) by panting against an occluded mouthpiece. If there is a lot of gas in the thorax, the swings in box pressure (A) compared to mouth pressure (B) will be much greater than if the lungs are small.

This is seen irrespective of whether the gas is in communication with the mouth, so poorly ventilated areas are measured. Abdominal gas can also influence the results, leading to a slight overestimation of thoracic gas volume. In normal subjects or those without airway disease, these two techniques yield similar results. With increasing severity of airflow obstruction, helium dilution tends to underestimate lung volumes, whereas plethysmography overestimates them[3].

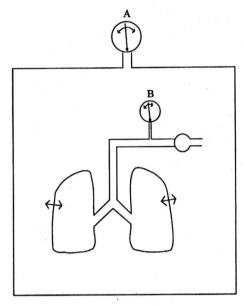

Figure 6.2

Comparison of lung volumes measured by both methods can sometimes be useful, as in this patient with a large bulla on his CXR:

PATIENT 6.07

Sex:	Female	Height (m):	1.71
Age (yrs):	49	Weight (kg):	65
Tobacco:	Ex-smoker	BMI (kg/m²):	22

	Measured	*% Predicted*	*SR*
Spirometry:			
FEV1 (L)	.55	20	-5.73
VC (L)	1.81	57	-3.17
FEV1/VC (%)	30	38	-7.38
Lung Volumes: (Helium dilution)			
RV (L)	2.28	114	+0.82
FRC (L)	3.03	105	+0.32
TLC (L)	4.33	79	-1.86
Lung Volumes: (Plethysmography)			
TGV (L)	5.89		
RV (L)	4.58	220	+3.22
FRC (L)	5.20	166	+1.96
TLC (L)	6.81	124	+1.27

The larger volumes by the plethysmographic method indicate that there is some gas which is not accessed during helium dilution, and give us an idea of the volume of the bulla.

(TGV stands for thoracic gas volume - this is the volume of air in the thorax at the time when the plethysmographic measurements were made. It may be different from FRC if the subject either inhales or exhales before starting to pant, or if the measurements are deliberately made at a different lung volume).

Plethysmography also provides an additional index of airflow obstruction, namely airways resistance. Not surprisingly, this is critically dependant on the lung volume at which it is measured - the airways are much wider open at TLC than they are at RV. Airways resistance should therefore be corrected for lung volume. For reasons we don't need to go into, the function of the airways is usually expressed as the reciprocal of resistance, which is called "conductance". "Specific conductance" is conductance corrected for lung volume, abbreviated to SGaw:

PATIENT 6.08

Sex:	Male		Height (m):	1.91
Age (yrs):	47		Weight (kg):	62
Tobacco:	Smoker		BMI (kg/m²):	17

	Measured	% Predicted	SR
Spirometry:			
FEV1 (L)	4.21	96	-0.31
VC (L)	5.27	96	-0.29
FEV1/VC (%)	80	97	-0.16
Lung Volumes: (Plethysmography)			
TGV (L)	6.42		
RV (L)	3.26	144	+1.31
FRC (L)	5.78	138	+1.11
TLC (L)	8.18	99	-0.02
SGaw (/kPa/s)	0.15		

SGaw can detect mild airflow obstruction when spirometry is normal, and can be used as a sensitive means of detecting bronchodilator response. Its utility is however limited by poor reproducibility, and the normal range quoted is derived from a comparatively small number of subjects[4]. The lower limit of the normal range for females is 1.04 /kPa/s and for males is 0.85 /kPa/s.

MIXED OBSTRUCTIVE/RESTRICTIVE DEFECTS

When we were analysing spirometry data without the benefit of full lung volumes, we decided that is was impossible to diagnose concomitant obstruction and restriction, since a low VC may be seen with either defect. In an obstructive defect we have already seen how TLC tends to be elevated. If it is normal, does this mean that there is superimposed restriction? How would you interpret these tests?

PATIENT 6.09

Sex:	Female		Height (m):	1.48
Age (yrs):	70		Weight (kg):	64
Tobacco:	Non-smoker		BMI (kg/m^2):	29

	Measured	% Predicted	SR
Spirometry:			
FEV1 (L)	0.60	40	-2.36
VC (L)	1.05	57	-1.85
FEV1/VC (%)	57	75	-2.87
Lung Volumes: (Helium dilution)			
RV (L)	2.64	147	+2.40
FRC (L)	2.75	115	+0.73
TLC (L)	3.69	93	-0.58

This patient clearly has airflow obstruction with a reduced FEV1/VC on spirometry. Her RV is high, but why is TLC not elevated as well? It is difficult to predict how much TLC will be elevated in airflow obstruction, and the interpretation depends on which technique was used to measure the volumes. We noted right at the start of this chapter that Helium dilution tends to underestimate lung volumes in the presence of airflow obstruction, and a normal TLC by this method is a very poor discriminator of additional restriction[5,6]. If TLC is low, we might cautiously suggest that there might be something else going on. Plethysmography, on the other hand, tends to overestimate TLC. A normal TLC by this latter method in the presence of what otherwise looks like airflow obstruction probably does lead us to *"Mixed restrictive and obstructive defect"*.

Elevation of RV is a much more consistent finding in airflow obstruction, so if this is normal or reduced we can infer with much more confidence that there are two processes taking place. Patient 6.10 had been a heavy smoker in the past, and presented with increasing breathlessness over a period of one year. He had fine crackles on auscultation of his lungs and his CXR showed diffuse reticulonodular shadowing:

PATIENT 6.10

Sex:	Male	Height (m):	1.72
Age (yrs):	70	Weight (kg):	66
Tobacco:	Ex-smoker	BMI (kg/m²):	22

	Measured	% Predicted	SR
Spirometry:			
FEV1 (L)	1.61	56	-2.49
VC (L)	4.60	123	+1.39
FEV1/VC (%)	35	47	-5.52
Lung Volumes: (Helium dilution)			
RV (L)	2.62	102	+0.15
FRC (L)	4.55	128	+1.65
TLC (L)	7.22	108	+0.80

Spirometry clearly shows a severe obstructive problem, and with an FEV1/VC of less than 50% we would expect to see an RV at least twice the predicted value[6]. This is not the case, so we can infer *"Mixed restrictive and obstructive defect"* with rather more confidence than if only TLC was not as high as expected.

Looking at mixed restrictive/obstructive patterns from the opposite angle, in a restrictive process we would expect RV, FRC and TLC all to be low. If in an otherwise restrictive picture the RV is elevated and the FEV/VC is low, then there is an obstructive element[7]. An example of this is in a patient with fibrosing alveolitis who has been a moderate smoker in previous years.

AIR TRAPPING AND RV/TLC (%)

In many sets of lung function test results RV is expressed in absolute terms and also as a percentage of TLC. The implication is that an elevated RV/TLC ratio reflects air trapping, although this term can also be applied to an elevated RV in isolation. Let's look at two examples:

	Measured	% Predicted	SR
PATIENT 6.04			
RV/TLC (%)	55	167	+4.08
PATIENT 6.11			
RV/TLC (%)	49	205	+4.64

Patient 6.04 is our earlier example of airflow obstruction, and so it not surprising that the RV/TLC ratio is high. If we rely on this index alone, we would also say that the other patient had airflow obstruction, but this proves to be incorrect when we look at all of the available data:

PATIENT 6.11

Sex:	Male	Arm span (m):	1.76
Age (yrs):	26	Weight (kg):	84
Tobacco:	Non-smoker	BMI (kg/m²):	27

	Measured	*% Predicted*	*SR*
Spirometry:			
FEV1 (L)	2.90	68	-2.71
VC (L)	3.15	62	-3.14
FEV1/VC (%)	92	111	+1.33
Lung Volumes: (Helium dilution)			
RV (L)	3.07	188	+3.50
FRC (L)	3.71	115	+0.79
TLC (L)	6.21	90	-1.15

As you can see from the spirometry, there is no suggestion of airflow obstruction. In fact the patient had a cervical spine transection: the reason RV is elevated is because the expiratory muscles are weak, and cannot compress the ribcage much below its resting level (hence the small difference between FRC and RV). Other causes of a relatively high RV are a stiff ribcage which is difficult to compress (as in ankylosing spondylitis or scoliosis) and chronic heart failure, when engorgement of the lungs with blood tends to act as a splint. Clearly this index is not specific to airflow obstruction; although it is sometimes useful (provided it is compared with the predicted value), for the sake of simplicity I have not included it in our reports.

SUMMARY

☞ In restrictive lung disease, lung volumes show a low FRC, RV and TLC. They may be abnormal even when spirometry is normal.

☞ In airflow obstruction, these volumes are usually elevated, particularly RV. A high RV/TLC ratio is also seen in some restrictive patterns.

☞ In the presence of an obstructive defect, a low TLC measured by helium dilution does not necessarily indicate an additional restrictive process.

☞ Plethysmography measures ventilated and unventilated gas, so can be used to assess the size of a bulla.

☞ A low Specific Conductance (SGaw) implies airflow obstruction.

REFERENCES

1. Owens MW, Kinasewitz GT, Anderson WM. Clinical significance of an isolated reduction in residual volume. *Am Rev Respir Dis* 1987;**136**:1377–1380.

2. Vulterini S, Bianco MR, Pellicciotti L, Sidoti AM. Lung mechanics in subjects showing increased residual volume without bronchial obstruction. *Thorax* 1980;**35**:461–466.

3. Rodenstein DO, Stanescu DC. Reassessment of lung volume measurement by helium and by body plethysography in chronic airflow obstruction. *Am Rev Respir Dis* 1982;**126**:1040–1044

4. Quanjer Ph. Standardized lung function testing. *Bull Europ Pathophysiol Respir* 1983;**19** (suppl 5):9

5. Barnhart S, Hudson LD, Mason SE, Pierson DJ, Rosenstock L. Total lung capacity. An insensitive measure of impairment in patients with asbestosis and chronic obstructive lung disease? *Chest* 1988;**93**:299–302.

6.   Lanier RC, Olsen GN. Can concomitant restriction be detected in adult men with airflow obstruction. *Chest* 1991;**99**:826–830.

7.   Schwartz DA, Merchant RK, Helmers RA, Gilbert SR, Dayton CS, Hunninghake GW. The influence of cigarette smoking on lung function in patients with idiopathic pulmonary fibrosis. *Am Rev Respir Dis* 1991;**144**:504–506.

7: GAS TRANSFER

Measurement of lung volumes is often combined with an assessment of gas transfer. Transfer of oxygen from inspired air into the circulation is what really matters physiologically, but carbon monoxide behaves in a similar fashion to oxygen in this process, and for technical reasons it is much easier to use carbon monoxide as the test gas. (Nitric oxide has some advantages over carbon monoxide, but is not yet in widespread use.)

The most commonly used technique is the single breath method, whereby the subject inhales the test gas, which contains a small concentration of carbon monoxide, and then holds their breath for ten seconds. Carbon monoxide is transported down to the alveoli by bulk movement, it then diffuses across the alveolar air space, through the alveolar lining cells and into the adjacent capillaries. Once in the blood, the carbon monoxide passes into red blood cells and combines with haemoglobin (Figure 7.1). When the subject breathes out, the amount of carbon monoxide remaining in the expired gas is measured (after disgarding the dead space volume): if the lungs are working well, most of the carbon monoxide will have combined with haemoglobin and there will be little left in the expirate. If there is a problem at any stage in the process of gas transfer, the carbon monoxide concentration in the expired gas will be much nearer to that of the test gas which was inspired.

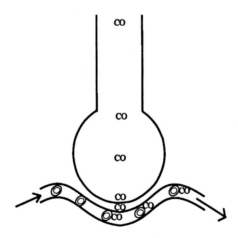

Figure 7.1

The following results were obtained from a patient suspected of having fibrosing alveolitis:

PATIENT 7.01

Sex	Female	Height (m)	1.58
Age (yrs)	58	Weight (kg)	81
Tobacco	Smoker	BMI (kg/m²)	32

	Measured	*% Predicted*	*SR*
Gas Transfer: (CO single breath, Hb=14.5 g/dl)			
TLCO (SI)	7.11	98	-0.13
KCO (SI)	2.03	101	+0.03

TLCO is short for "transfer factor" (Transfer factor for the Lung for Carbon monOxide), and gives in indication of the total ability of the lungs to transfer this gas across into the bloodstream. The SI units of measurement are mmol/min/kPa.

KCO stands for transfer coefficient. It is calculated by dividing TLCO by lung volume (alveolar volume, to be precise). KCO is expressed as mmol/min/kPa/L (to save space the units for TLCO and CCO are abbreviated to "SI" in subsequent examples). We'll look at the differences between TLCO and KCO in different diseases later in this chapter.

(The ERS recommendations give a prediction equation for TLCO[1], which I have used; at the time of writing there is still debate about how to calculate predicted KCO[2]. Predicted TLCO/predicted TLC can be used, but we do not have an RSD for this method to use in defining our normal range. I have therefore used the equations given by Cotes in Lung Function[3].)

You may have noticed that the haemoglobin concentration is given with the results. When carbon monoxide has passed through the lungs into the pulmonary capillaries, if there aren't many red cells present then the amount of haemoglobin available for it to bind to will be less and as a consequence TLCO and KCO will be low.

The importance of correcting TLCO and KCO for the haemoglobin concentration is illustrated in the next patient who presented with breathlessness on exertion. His gas transfer results, calculated if we assume his haemoglobin concetration is normal, are as follows:

PATIENT 7.02A

Sex	Male	Height (m)	1.83
Age (yrs)	23	Weight (kg)	50
Tobacco	Non-smoker	BMI (kg/m^2)	15

	Measured	% Predicted	SR
Gas Transfer: (CO single breath, Hb=14.5 g/dl)			
TLCO (51)	.92	46	-4.75
KCO (51)	1.04	61	-2.41

The low TLCO and KCO might lead us to think that his lungs are abnormal. In fact he has a severe iron deficiency anaemia, with a haemoglobin of 4.8 g/dl. When we correct for this in our calculations, his results look quite different:

PATIENT 7.02B

Sex:	Male	Height (m):	1.83
Age (yrs):	23	Weight (kg):	50
Tobacco:	Non-smoker	BMI (kg/m^2):	15

	Measured	% Predicted	SR
Gas Transfer: (CO single breath, Hb=4.8 g/dl)			
TLCO (51)	10.87	85	-1.26
KCO (51)	1.90	99	-0.04

If the haemoglobin concentration is not known, gas transfer data should be interpreted with caution.

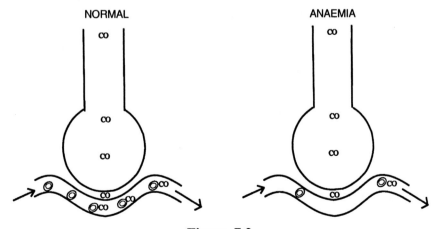

Figure 7.2

When the alveolar-capillary membrane is thickened, as in a patient with fibrosing alveolitis, the distance which the test gas has to travel to reach the blood is increased, TLCO and KCO will be low:

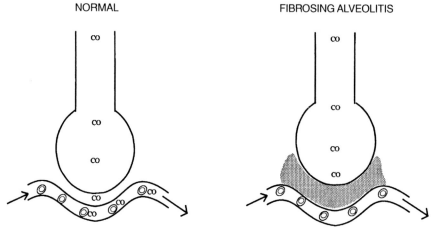

NORMAL   FIBROSING ALVEOLITIS

Figure 7.3

PATIENT 7.03

Sex:	Male	Height (m):	1.78
Age (yrs):	47	Weight (kg):	65
Tobacco:	Non-smoker	BMI (kg/m²):	20

	Measured	*% Predicted*	*SR*
Spirometry:			
FEV1 (L)	1.80	38	-4.78
VC (L)	1.50	39	-4.57
FEV1/VC (%)	83	105	+0.61
Lung Volumes: (Helium dilution)			
RV (L)	1.51	72	-1.47
FRC (L)	2.47	71	-1.70
TLC (L)	3.31	46	-6.39
Gas Transfer: (CO single breath, Hb=15.3 g/dl)			
TLCO (SI)	2.99	28	-5.46
KCO (SI)	0.91	47	-3.77

There is clearly a restrictive defect, but with the gas transfer data we can now comment on the function of the lungs. TLCO is reduced, so the overall ability to transfer gas is reduced. This is not just a reflection of the fact that the lungs are small, since KCO is also low (see below). Our report should be *"Severe restrictive defect with impaired gas transfer"*.

The combination of a restrictive ventilatory defect with low TLCO and KCO is seen in many diseases which cause inflammation or fibrosis of the alveoli. (There is some evidence that TLCO and KCO increase in the very early "alveolitic" phase of some of these diseases[4], one suggestion being that the alveolar-capillary membrane is "leaky" and allows carbon monoxide to pass through paracellular channels.)

We have already noted the effect of anaemia on gas transfer. A similar problem arises when the amount of blood flowing through the pulmonary capillaries is low, for example in a patient with pulmonary vasculitis:

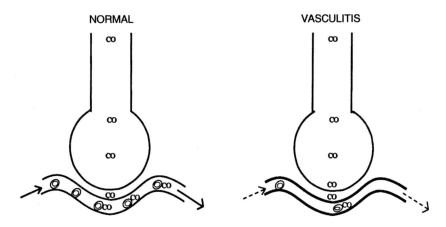

Figure 7.4

PATIENT 7.04

Sex:	Female	Height (m):	1.59
Age (yrs):	71	Weight (kg):	49
Tobacco:	Non-smoker	BMI (kg/m²):	19

	Measured	*% Predicted*	*SR*
Spirometry:			
FEV1 (L)	1.90	99	-0.03
VC (L)	2.65	114	+0.79
FEV1/VC (%)	72	95	-0.60
Lung Volumes: (Helium dilution)			
RV (L)	1.51	75	-1.43
FRC (L)	2.38	90	-0.50
TLC (L)	4.16	88	-0.90
Gas Transfer: (CO single breath, Hb=14.1 g/dl)			
TLCO (SI)	2.49	41	-3.42
KCO (SI)	0.65	41	-4.60

Note that the lung volumes are normal but that TLCO and KCO are low. (It might be prudent to check that the haemoglobin concentration is correct.) A similar picture is seen in pulmonary embolism or when a right-to-left intra-cardiac shunt results in pulmonary oligaemia. Failure to realise that TLCO and KCO depend not only on the state of the alveoli but also on pulmonary blood flow is a common misunderstanding. These indices give an assessment of how the surface area of normal alveolar surface is in contact with functioning circulation.

TLCO and KCO are sensitive tests of pulmonary function, and may be the first to become impaired when the alveoli are abnormal. For example, a low TLCO and KCO in an immunocompromised patient can point to the possibility of pneumocystis infection, at a time when the chest X-ray and lung volumes are normal. Our report of Patient 7.04 should encompass all these possibilities: *"Normal lung volumes but impaired gas transfer. A pulmonary vascular problem is the most likely explanation, although an early alveolitic or fibrotic process should also be considered. (Please check that the haemoglobin concentration is correct, since these results would fit with anaemia)."*

EXTRA-PULMONARY RESTRICTION

In the examples we have looked at so far, TLCO and KCO have both been reduced. We now need to consider why they might change in different directions. If you were to measure my transfer factor, you would ask me to take a deep breath in from RV to TLC, with the following results:

	Measured	*% Predicted*	*SR*
TLCO (SI)	12.7	110	+0.88
KCO (SI)	1.73	111	+0.69

Look at what happens if instead I only take a small breath in, say from RV up to about FRC. Because my lungs are not fully inflated, the surface area available for gas exchange is lower than it should be and TLCO is low:

	Measured	*% Predicted*	*SR*
TLCO (51)	6.44	56	-3.54

If my cardiac output remains the same, the same volume of blood has to get through the lungs somehow. The density of blood per unit lung volume is therefore higher, with distension of the pulmonary capillaries. The result is that my KCO is high:

	Measured	% Predicted	SR
KCO	3.04	196	+5.73

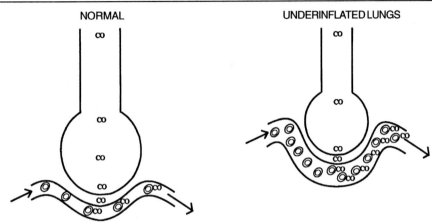

Figure 7.5

In patients with a restrictive ventilatory defect caused by an extra-pulmonary problem (e.g. muscle weakness, scoliosis, pleural disease) KCO will therefore be elevated:

PATIENT 7.05

Sex:	Male	Height (m):	1.86
Age (yrs):	17	Weight (kg):	56
Tobacco:	Non-smoker	BMI (kg/m²):	16

	Measured	% Predicted	SR
Spirometry:			
FEV1 (L)	2.15	43	-5.62
VC (L)	2.30	39	-5.95
FEV1/VC (%)	93	111	+1.30
Lung Volumes: (Helium dilution)			
RV (L)	1.23	78	-0.86
FRC (L)	2.09	61	-2.21
TLC (L)	3.53	45	-7.09
Gas Transfer: (CO single breath, Hb=14.1 g/dl)			
TLCO (SI)	8.98	66	-3.20
KCO (SI)	2.74	121	+1.83

The restrictive defect with low TLCO is similar to the pattern we saw in Patient 7.04, although the preservation of RV would lead us to suspect a stiff chest wall or weak expiratory muscles (see chapter 6). The high KCO tells us that the ability of the lungs to transfer gas is probably fine when we take their size into account.

A similar pattern with a low TLCO but high KCO is seen after pneumonectomy, when all the cardiac output is passing through one lung - a common example used in textbooks and exam questions. However interesting this might be physiologically, it is often easier to ask the patient if they have had a lung removed rather than infer it from lung function tests.

At the start if this chapter we noted that KCO is calculated by dividing TLCO by alveolar volume. A common misconception is that KCO is therefore an indication of gas transfer per unit of lung volume, irrespective of the size of the lungs. KCO does vary with lung volume, as we have seen, mainly because of the corresponding changes in the density of blood per unit of lung volume. Gas transfer results must therefore be looked at in the light of the size of the lungs, as indicated by TLC or by alveolar volume if the latter is given separately. Some suggestions have been made as to how this effect can be allowed for[5], but are not yet in widespread use.

AIRFLOW OBSTRUCTION

If the carbon monoxide in the inspired gas is delivered to the mouth of an emphysematous airspace, it has a longer distance to diffuse before it reaches the alveolar lining cells:

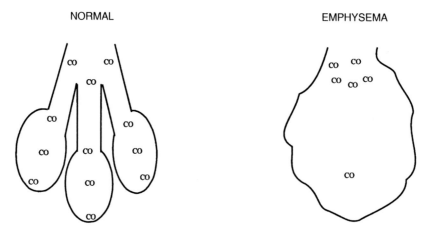

Figure 7.6

The total surface area available for gas exchange is also reduced, so TLCO (and KCO) will be low:

PATIENT 7.06

Sex:	Male	Height (m):	1.73
Age (yrs):	44	Weight (kg):	59
Tobacco:	Smoker	BMI (kg/m^2):	20

	Measured	*% Predicted*	*SR*
Spirometry:			
FEV1 (L)	2.40	34	-2.50
VC (L)	4.25	95	-0.38
FEV1/VC (%)	56	71	-3.18
Lung Volumes: (Helium dilution)			
RV (L)	2.91	145	+2.21
FRC (L)	5.22	156	+3.11
TLC (L)	7.16	106	+0.70
Gas Transfer: (CO single breath, Hb=16.2 g/dl)			
TLCO (51)	4.30	42	-4.23
KCO (51)	0.59	30	-5.03

If we only had transfer factor to go on, it would be difficult to say what the underlying pathology was. However, the lung volumes show an obstructive pattern, and emphysema is much the most likely diagnosis (with TLC being underestimated by helium dilution).

In asthma, TLCO and/or KCO may be elevated, particularly if TLC is high. Debate continues about the exact cause of this increase; some of it may be to do with the technicalities of performing a single-breath transfer factor in a patient with airflow obstruction[6]. Hyperaemia of the airways probably also contributes, with carbon monoxide binding to red blood cells in vessels along the airways. In the upright posture, perfusion of the lung apices may also be greater in patients with asthma than in a normal subject, similar to the pattern seen during exercise, which may increase gas transfer[7].

PATIENT 7.07

Sex	Female	Height (m)	1.54
Age (yrs)	52	Weight (kg)	75
Tobacco	Smoker	BMI (kg/m²)	32

	Measured	% Predicted	SR
Spirometry:			
FEV1 (L)	1.05	48	-2.98
VC (L)	2.15	83	-1.00
FEV1/VC (%)	70	89	-1.45
Lung Volumes: (Helium dilution)			
RV (L)	2.45	151	+2.37
FRC (L)	2.73	109	+0.46
TLC (L)	4.60	105	+0.45
Gas Transfer (CO single breath, Hb=12.8 g/dl)			
TLCO (SI)	9.67	132	+2.02
KCO (SI)	2.10	103	+0.13

This brings us to the question of "effective" transfer factor. In the calculation of single breath TLCO, two different volumes can be used. The more usual volume is RV, as measured beforehand by rebreathing helium dilution or plethysmography. The alternative method is to use the alveolar volume (VA) which is accessed during the single breath manoeuvre itself, inferred from dilution of helium in the test gas mixture. In restrictive lung disease, the two volumes are usually similar. However, if there is significant airflow obstruction, VA estimated from a single breath may be much smaller than RV measured when several minutes are allowed for equilibration of helium during the rebreathing test, or using plethysmography which does not depend on gas dilution.

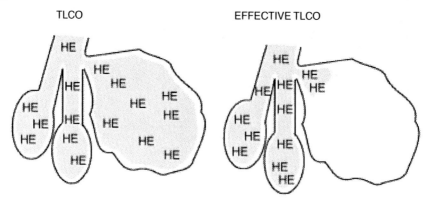

Figure 7.7

TLCO calculated using VA is known as the "effective" TLCO. The adjective "effective" is used, since this is the volume of lung to which there is access during the ten second breath hold - a larger volume might be accesible with longer equilibration times, but these "slower" parts of the lung contribute little to overall alveolar ventilation during normal respiration. Moreover, we are probably not justified in assuming that the lung which is not accessed during the ten-second breath holding time will have the same gas transfer properties as that which we have actually measured.

Effective TLCO may be very much lower than TLCO in patients with severe airflow obstruction, even when there is no emphysema:

PATIENT 7.08

Sex:	Male	Height (m):	1.83
Age (yrs):	41	Weight (kg):	66
Tobacco:	Smoker	BMI (kg/m²):	20

	Measured	*% Predicted*	*SR*
Spirometry:			
FEV1 (L)	1.50	36	-5.27
VC (L)	4.00	78	-1.85
FEV1/VC (%)	37	47	-5.90
Lung Volumes: (Helium dilution)			
RV (L)	3.62	175	+3.78
FRC (L)	5.01	141	+2.42
TLC (L)	7.62	101	+0.11
Gas Transfer (CO single breath, Hb=13.4 g/dl)			
TLCO (SI)	7.07	61	-3.21
Effective TLCO (SI)	5.20	45	-4.54
KCO (SI)	0.98	55	-2.96

These differences are interesting but seldom of much importance in clinical practice.

INCREASED GAS TRANSFER

As you might expect, an excess of haemoglobin available for carbon monoxide to bind to leads to an increased transfer factor. Carbon monoxide will combine with haemoglobin wherever it encounters it, so if there has been haemorrhage into the lung TLCO and KCO will be increased[8]:

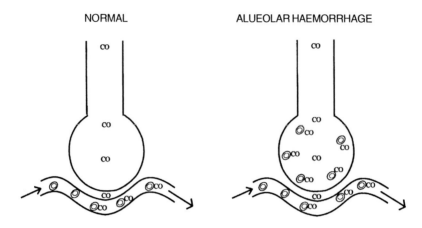

NORMAL   ALUEOLAR HAEMORRHAGE

Figure 7.8

Serial mesurement of gas transfer can be used to monitor the progress of intra-pulmonary hammorrhage, as in this patient with Wegener's granulomatosis who presented with a flare up of his disease on 17th December 1996. The following day he became breathless and a CXR showed bilateral diffuse infiltrates. Baseline data from one year previously were available for comparison.

PATIENT 7.09

Sex:	Male		Height (m):	1.7
Age (yrs):	38		Weight (kg):	76
Tobacco:	Non-smoker		BMI (kg/m²):	26

Date	Hb g/dl	TLCO mmol/kPa/min	% pred	SR
27/4/95	14.6	9.4	90	-0.80
17/12/96	12.2	10.8	104	+0.32
19/12/96	10.4	12.8	123	+1.69
23/12/96	10.2	19.6	188	+6.47
27/12/96	12.1	11.7	113	+0.97

The abrupt increase in TLCO is characteristic of pulmonary haemorrhage, which also explains the drop in Hb. An increase in transfer factor can be seen in polycythaemia, or if the pulmonary capillaries are distended by a left-to-right shunt.

SUMMARY

☞ A low TLCO and KCO can be caused by anaemia, emphysema, pulmonary oedema, alveolitis, fibrosis, right-to-left shunts and pulmonary vascular disease.

☞ A high TLCO and KCO can be the result of pulmonary haemorrhage, polycythaemia or left-to-right shunting.

☞ In a pulmonary restrictive process, the TLCO and KCO should be low; if the TLCO is low and the KCO normal or high, suspect extra-pulmonary restriction.

☞ With airflow obstruction, a low TLCO implies emphysema. In asthma the TLCO is often high.

REFERENCES

1. Cotes JE, Chinn DJ, Quanjer PhH, Roca J, Yernault J-C. Standardisation of the measurement of transfer factor (diffusing capacity). *Eur Respir J* 1993;**6**(Suppl 16):41–53.

2. Love RG, Seaton A. About the ECCS summary equations. *Eur Respir J* 1990;3:489.

3. Cotes J. *Lung function*. Blackwell, Oxford 1993.

4. Dujic Z, Tocilj J, Eterovic D. Increase of lung transfer factor in early sarcoidosis. *Resp Med* 1995,**89**:9–14.

5. Chinn DJ, Cotes JE, Flowers R, Marks A-M, Reed JW. Transfer factor (diffusing capacity) standardized for alveolar volume: validation, refernce values and applications of a new linear model to replace KCO (TL/VA). *Eur Respir J* 1996;**9**:1269–1277.

6. Keens TG, Mansell A, Krastins IRB, Levison H, Bryon AC, Hyland RH, Zamel N. Evaluation of the single breath diffusing capacity in asthma and cystic fibrosis. *Chest* 1979;**76**:41–44.

7.   Weitzman RG, Wilson AF. Diffusing capacity and overall ventilation:perfusion in asthma. *Am J Med* 1974;**57**:767–774.

8.   Lipscomb DJ, Patel K, Hughes JMB. Interpretation of increases in the transfer coeficient for carbon monoxide (Tlco/VA or Kco). *Thorax* 1979;**33**:728–733.

8: "CONSISTENT WITH THE DIAGNOSIS OF ..."

Lung function tests are sometimes requested on a "Breathless - ? cause" basis. Even without much clinical information, we can sometimes make suggestions as to possible underlying diagnoses in our report, if the results fit a typical pattern, for example of emphysema.

Not infrequently, the request is more along the lines of "We know this patient has Disease X, but are their lungs involved?" or "We know this patient has Disease Y, but is there anything else going on to explain their breathlessness?". With these other scenarios in mind, the rest of this chapter outlines some patterns of lung function tests which are seen in the more common respiratory diseases, with some rarer ones we might occassionally encounter. I have only included those diseases where I think the information will be of use in reporting lung function tests.

You might wonder why I've included some topics: for example, there are other ways of diagnosing a pleural effusion than from lung function tests! However, it might be useful to know whether the lung function tests of a patient with a small pleural effusion suggest that there is additional pulmonary disease. In order to decide this, we need to know what the presence of pleural fluid does to lung function test results.

One other justification of my choice of diseases is that this is not meant to be a textbook of respiratory medicine - the associations of fibrosing alveolitis, for example, are well dealt with elsewhere and scleroderma, ulcerative colitis, primary biliary cirrhosis, etc. don't get a separate mention. Where a pattern of respiratory abnormality is common to several different diseases (pulmonary vasculitis or haemorrhage, for example), I have described the abnormality only once rather than list it repeatedly under each disease.

This is not meant to be a comprehensive account of all that is known about pulmonary function in every disease, but I've given rather more references than in previous chapters. I've usually stuck to one reference, whenever possible, in an easily accesible journal. Bates (see "Bibliography") has over 5000 references if you need to look further afield.

"CLASSICAL" RESPIRATORY DISEASES

We have already discussed these topics in some detail in previous chapters, but it will do no harm to re-cap.

Asthma

By definition, asthma is associated with an obstructive defect on spirometry. As we've already discussed, an elevated RV is common as the result of premature airway closure during expiration, and may be the only abnormality in mild cases. Elevation of TLC is seen in more severe asthma, and in such cases the TLCO (and/or the KCO) may also be elevated, possibly reflecting airway inflammation with CO binding to red cells in vessels in airways[1,2].

Bronchiectasis

Bronchiectasis also causes airflow obstruction, but the fibrotic component of the disease process means that TLC and RV are low. Destruction of lung tissue would normally lower transfer factor, but airway inflammation exerts an opposing effect (as in asthma), so that TLCO is only slightly low and KCO is normal[3].

Chronic obstructive airways disease

COAD, like asthma, by definition is associated with an obstructive defect. (By COAD, or COPD if you prefer, I mean chronic bronchitis with airflow obstruction. Emphysema is considered separately). Premature airway closure during expiration means that RV is commonly elevated. TLC should also be elevated, and often is when measured plethysmographically, although the helium dilution technique may generate spuriously low values in patients with severe airflow obstruction. The TLCO and KCO are normal in COAD (in contrast to emphysema) although the "effective" TLCO may be low (see previous chapter).

Emphysema

Emphysema is associated with an obstructive defect on spirometry. Loss of lung tissue means that inward elastic recoil is less than normal, and airways close prematurely during expiration; both these factors lead to elevation of RV, which can be very marked. TLC is often normal when measured by helium dilution; as ever in the presence of severe airflow obstruction, TLC by plethysmography may be greater than by helium dilution in more severe cases. A discrepancy between the two techniques is a pointer to the presence of poorly ventilated bullae. In early disease, an elevated RV may be the only abnormality. Poor bulk transfer of air to the alveoli, and reduced surface area for gas exchange means that TLCO and KCO are low.

Extrinsic allergic alveolitis

Inflammation of alveoli impairs gas exchange, so TLCO and KCO are often markedly reduced. Stiffness of the lungs causes a mild restrictive defect, with low TLC and VC. However, involvment of bronchioles may cause an element of obstruction with low FEV1/VC ratio and relatively well preserved RV[4].

Fibrosing alveolitis

Classically fibrosing alveolitis causes a restrictive defect, reflecting stiffness of the lungs, but in the early stages this may only be seen on full lung volumes. Thickening of the alveolar-capillary membrane leads to reduction of both TLCO and KCO[5].

Pneumoconiosis

In comparison with a patient with fibrosing alveolitis who has radiographic shadowing of similar severity, pulmonary function in someone with pneumoconiosis is often surprisingly normal. In more severe cases fibrosis develops and there is a restrictive defect. Similarly, any reduction in TLCO and KCO tends to be small. Airflow obstruction is seen in coal-workers' pneumoconiosis, particularly if the patient is a smoker as well. Asbestosis is associated with the typical pattern of a restrictive defect, with slightly low TLCO and KCO[6], although in the early "alveolitic" stages there is some suggestion that TLCO and KCO may be high[7]. One possible explanation for this early rise in transfer factor is "leakiness" of the alveolar-capillary membrane, allowing CO easier passage into the blood vessels. Diffuse pleural disease can also cause restriction with a low TLCO, but the KCO is then high[8]. The occurrence of airflow obstruction with asbestos exposure is controversial[9].

Specific pneumoconioses are covered in more detail in textbooks dedicated to this subject[10,11].

Pulmonary embolism

Undiagnosed pulmonary embolic disease is probably quite a common explanation for breathlessness in patients referred to the lung function laboratory for assessment. Lung volumes are usually normal, although recurrent infarction can lead to fibrosis and a mild restrictive pattern. TLCO and KCO may be slightly reduced if there is significant disruption of pulmonary blood flow, but are often surprisingly normal[12,13].

Sarcoidosis

Fibrotic sarcoidosis causes a restrictive defect, usually with low TLCO and KCO[14]. As with asbestos exposure, there is some suggestion that TLCO and KCO may be high in the early phases of the disease[15]. Airflow obstruction is also seen fairly commonly[16], as a consequence of airway inflammation and scarring.

OTHER FAIRLY COMMON PROBLEMS

AIDS

TLCO (and KCO) are often the first lung function tests to become abnormal, particularly with opportunistic infections such as pneumocystis, with a restrictive defect developing later if alveolar damage progresses to fibrosis[17]. Airflow obstruction is occassionally seen with endobronchial Kaposi lesions[18].

Allergic broncho-pulmonary aspergillosis

Rather like other causes of bronchiectasis, there is an obstructive defect with a high RV, but TLC is normal or even reduced because of the fibrotic component of the the disease. TLCO and KCO are usually normal[19].

Ankylosing spondylitis

Immobility of the chest wall means that it is difficult for the inspiratory muscles to inflate the thorax to a normal TLC, and equally for the expiratory muscles to deflate it down to a normal RV. Thus TLC is low, but RV is normal or even high. TLCO is low since the lungs at TLC are smaller than normal, so, therefore, is the surface area available for gas exchange, but congestion of these small lungs means that KCO is high - a classical "extrapulmonary" restriction[20]. If pulmonary fibrosis develops, TLC and TLCO are further reduced and KCO becomes normal or even reduced.

Arterio-venous malformations

Lung volumes are usually normal, but TLCO and KCO are low because of shunting of blood through the abnormal vascular channels, which means that there is less blood in the alveolar capillaries for carbon monoxide to combine with[21].

Ascites

Ascites causes remarkably little change in lung volumes, apart from a small reduction in FRC[22]. TLCO and KCO are normal.

Bone Marrow Transplantation

In the first few months after bone marrow transplantation, there is a mild restrictive defect with low TLCO and KCO. This probably reflects damage by cytotoxic drugs to the alveoli, and there is some improvement up to about 12 months. The picture of bronchiolitis obliterans (see below) supervenes if graft-versus-host disease develops[23].

Bronchiolitis obliterans

Bronchiolitis obliterans organising pneumonia, or BOOP, means different things to different people. The obstructive part of this disease process leads to a low FEV1 and FEV1/VC ratio, with an elevated RV, and this is the typical pattern seen in patients in whom the "bronchiolitis" component predominates. If there is much "obliterans", then a restrictive defect is seen, with TLCO and KCO both reduced[24]. This latter picture is that seen with the "organising pneumonia" part of the BOOP complex.

Cirrhosis

Lung volumes are normal in cirrhosis, but a low TLCO and KCO may be seen if there are pulmonary arterio-venous malformations[25], which divert blood away from gas exchanging tissue and thus reduce the amount of haemoglobin available to combine with CO.

Coronary artery by-pass graft

After thoracotomy there is a mild restrictive defect. The TLCO is low because the lungs are small, but as with other "extra-pulmonary" problems the KCO is normal[26].

Cystic fibrosis

Airflow obstruction is common, but the TLC may be low as a result of atelectasis[27]. TLCO is often surprisingly normal, although it may also be reduced if there is much lung destruction. The KCO is usually normal, even when the TLCO is reduced, perhaps because of airway inflammation, with CO combining with haemoglobin in blood vessels in airway walls[2].

Diabetes mellitus

TLCO and KCO are slightly low, probably because of thickening of the alveolar capillary membrane, but lung volumes are normal[28].

Drugs

Many drugs can affect the lungs, the most common abnormality being reduced TLCO and KCO reflecting alveolar damage. On withdrawal of the drug, recovery usually occurs over a period of up to 12 months, but some permanent damage may persist, for example after administration of cytotoxic agents[29].

Eosinophilic pneumonia

Pulmonary eosinophilia can be associated with several different diseases. Infiltration of the alveoli causes stiffness of the lungs, with a restrictive defect. Gas exchange is impaired by the presence of eosinophils, but also by any associated pulmonary vasulitis, so that TLCO and KCO are low. Airflow obstruction is common, even in patients who do not have an asthmatic history, reflecting the bronchiolitic component of the disease[30,31].

Heart failure

Pulmonary oedema makes the lungs stiff, so TLC and VC tend to be low, but airway oedema means that FEV1/VC may also be slightly low. As with other forms of pulmonary congestion, the distended vascular tree splints the lungs and so RV is often high. The effect of TLCO and KCO is variable, depending upon the balance between congestion, which increases the available haemoglobin, and oedema which tends to decrease carbon monoxide transfer. Chronic congestion can progress to fibrosis, which also reduces gas transfer[32].

Hemiplegia

There is surprisingly little data on lung function after a stroke. VC and TLC are low initially, with some recovery over a period of months.

Inflammatory bowel disease

Alveolar damage in patients with inflammatory bowel disease is quite common, and TLCO and KCO are often low even in the absence of respiratory symptoms, for reasons which are unclear. Classical fibrosing alveolitis and bronchiolitis may both be seen, more usually with ulcerative colitis.

Kyphosis

Kyphosis causes much less severe restriction than scoliosis. The restrictive defect mainly affects VC and TLC, with RV fairly well preserved[33]. TLCO is reduced but KCO is high. See also "Scoliosis".

Lobectomy

After lobectomy there is a mild reduction in all volumes, and consequently TLCO. KCO is normal, because of the increased amount of blood flowing through the remaining lung[34]. See also "Pneumonectomy".

Myopathy

The pattern of ventilatory defect in myopathies depends on the relative weakness of expiratory and inspiratory muscles. VC and TLC are low if the inspiratory muscles are weak, partly reflecting the weakness but also because the lungs become stiffer if they are chronically underventilated. RV tends to be normal or slightly high if the expiratory muscles are affected. TLCO is reduced because the lungs are small, but KCO is elevated, as with any extrapulmonary restriction[35].

Obesity

Restrictive defects are quite commonly attributed to obesity, but it is worth remembering that mild obesity (BMI 25-30) causes surprisingly little change in pulmonary function, apart from a slight reduction in FRC. This reduction in FRC becomes more marked as the obesity becomes more severe[36].

Organising pneumonitis

See "Bronchiolitis obliterans".

Parkinson's

Dysfunction of the respiratory muscles in this condition can lead to a mild restriction of lung volumes, but gas transfer is normal[37].

Pituitary disease

Underdevelopment of the lungs in hypopituitarism can cause TLC and VC to be low[38]. Lung function is otherwise normal. Excessive lung growth in long-standing acromegaly leads to a mild elevation of VC and TLC. Other volumes, TLCO and KCO are normal. Upper airway obstruction may occassionally be seen as a result of laryngeal abnormalities[39].

Pleural effusion

Pleural fluid expands the chest wall outwards rather more than it pushes the lungs inward, so any reduction in VC and TLC is less than might be expected from the volume of fluid present in the pleural space. Any reduction in lung size does however decrease TLCO, with a normal or high KCO[40].

Pneumonectomy

Lung volumes and TLCO are reduced after pneumonectomy, but generally only by about 30%. Since all the cardiac output passes through one lung, there is more haemoglobin available for CO to combine with and so KCO is high[34]. See also "Lobectomy".

Pneumothorax

Spirometry shows a restrictive pattern in patients with a pneumothorax. The pattern of lung volumes seen will depend upon whether plethysmography is used, in which case there will be little abnormality. Helium dilution will not measure the air in the pneumothorax, so the lung volumes will be reduced. TLCO may be slightly reduced, with a normal KCO, reflecting compression of the lungs[40].

Pregnancy

As pregnancy progresses, a restrictive defect develops but with a relatively high RV. There is little information about gas transfer, but TLCO and KCO probably remain normal or become slightly reduced[41].

Primary pulmonary hypertension

TLCO and KCO are reduced in primary pulmonary hypertension, because there is less blood flowing through the pulmonary vessels with which CO can combine. There may also be a mild restrictive defect[42].

Pulmonary haemorrhage

TLCO and KCO are high with any form of pulmonary haemorrhage, on account of the free availability of haemoglobin with which CO can combine[43]. Lung volumes are normal.

Radiation

Radiation causes an acute pneumonitis, which impairs gas transfer but with little effect on volumes. TLCO and KCO start to decline after a few months, but usually recover within one year. Fibrosis can lead to a mild residual restrictive defect[44].

Renal failure

TLCO and KCO may be reduced in patients with chronic renal failure, probably reflecting thickening of the alveolar capillary membrane[45]. Peritoneal dialysis causes a mild restrictive defect initially, with recovery to normal lung volumes within two weeks[46].

Scoliosis

The extrathoracic restriction of scoliosis leads to low lung volumes, but TLC and VC are affected more than RV on account of the ribcage being difficult to compress below FRC. TLCO is down because the lungs are small but the KCO is high[47].

Sickle cell disease

Sickle cell disease causes a slightly low TLC and VC, with low TLCO and KCO, for reasons which are unclear. The FEV1/VC ratio may also be low[48].

Thoracoplasty

The surgical treatment of tuberculosis almost invariably leads to loss of lung volume, but it was only resorted to in patients with extensive disease, in whom some endobronchial scarring is common. A mixed restrictive and obstructive pattern is therefore almost invariable. TLCO is usually reduced, but the KCO is normal[49].

Thyroid disease

The hyperdynamic circulatory state of hyperthyroidism causes pulmonary vascular congestion, with a high RV, low VC and TLC. The respiratory myopathy of hypothyroidism causes a low TLC and VC, with relatively normal RV. Lung function is otherwise normal[50].

Vasculitis

Disruption of flow through the pulmonary capillaries causes TLCO and KCO to be low when vasculitis affects the pulmonary vasculature. There may also be a mild restrictive defect.

SOME RARITIES

Alveolar microlithiasis

Lung function is often surprisingly normal in this condition, but it may progress to a restrictive defect with low TLCO and KCO as the alveoli become more abnormal[51].

Alveolar proteinosis

Lung volumes are normal or show mild restriction in alveolar proteinosis, but the proteinaceous material in the alveoli causes a low TLCO and KCO[52].

Amyloidosis

In amyloidosis lung function is usually normal, but depending upon the pattern of deposition there may also be a low TLCO and KCO with or without a restrictive defect. More rarely, endobronchial lesions can cause either generalized airflow obstruction, or large airway obstruction on a flow-volume loop[53].

Eosinophilic granuloma

Initially there is restrictive defect with low TLCO and KCO. In later stages an obstructive element may appear, with low FEV1/VC and elevated RV[54].

Haemosiderosis

Pulmonary haemosiderosis complicates a number of connective tissue diseases and vasculitides. Lungs volumes are normal but TLCO and KCO are elevated[43].

Lymphangioleiomyomatosis

Muscular changes in the airways cause an obstructive defect, with high RV and TLC[55]. The TLCO and KCO are low because of cystic changes with a reduction in the surface area available for gas exchange.

Neurofibromatosis

Fibrosis leads to a restrictive defect with low TLCO and KCO, but an obstructive picture may also be seen.

REFERENCES

1. Weitzman RG, Wilson AF. Diffusing capacity and overall ventilation:perfusion in asthma. *Am J Med* 1974;**57**:767–774.

2. Keens TG, Mansell A, Krastins IRB, Levison H, Bryon AC, Hyland RH, Zamel N. Evaluation of the single breath diffusing capacity in asthma and cystic fibrosis. *Chest* 1979;**76**:41–44.

3. Landau L, Phelan PD, Williams HE. Ventilatory mechanics in patients with bronchiectasis starting in childhood. *Thorax* 1974;**29**:304–312.

4. Warren CPW, Tse KS, Cherniak RM. Mechanical properties of the lung in extrinsic allergic alveolitis. *Thorax* 1978;**33**:315–321.

5. Agusti C, Xaubet A, Agusti AGN, Roca J, Ramirez J, Rodriguez-Rosin R. Clinical and functional assessment of patients with idiopathic pulmonary fibrosis: results of a 3 year follow-up. *Eur Respir J* 1994;**7**:643–650.

6. Markos J, Musk AW, Finucane KE. Functional similarities of asbestosis and cryptogenic fibrosing alveolitis. *Thorax* 1988;**43**:708–714.

7. Dujic Z, Tocilj J, Boschi S, Saric M, Eterovic D. Biphasic lung diffusing capacity: detection of early asbestos induced changes in lung function. *Br J Indust Med* 1992;**49**:260–267.

8. Yates DH, Browne K, Stidolph PN, Neville E. Asbestos-related bilateral diffuse pleural thickening: natural history of radiographic and lung function abnormalities. *Am J Respir Crit Care Med* 1996;**153**:301–306.

9. Kilburn KH, Warshaw RH. Airways obstruction from asbestos exposure and asbestosis revisited. *Chest* 1995;**107**:1730–1731.

10. Morgan WKC, Seaton A. *Occupational lung disorders*. WB Saunders, Philadelphia 1984.

11. Parkes WR. *Occupational lung disorders.* Butterworth-Heinemann, Oxford 1994.

12. Morris TA, Auger WR, Ysrael MZ, Olson LK, Channick RN, Fedullo PF, Moser KM.Parenchymal scarring is associated with restrictive spirometric defects in patients with chronic thromboembolic pulmonary hypertension. *Chest* 1996;**110**:399–403.

13. Wimalartna HSK, Farrell J, Lee HY. Measurement of diffusing capacity in pulmonary embolism. *Resp Med* 1989;**83**:481–485.

14. Marshall R, Karlish AJ. Lung function in sarcoidosis. *Thorax* 1971;26:402-405.

15. Dujic Z, Tocilj J, Eterovic D. Increase of lung transfer factor in early sarcoidosis. *Respiratory Medicine* 1995;**89**:9–14.

16. Sharma OM, Johnson RJ. Airway obstruction in sarcoidosis. *Chest* 1988;**94**:343–346.

17. Rosen MJ, Lou Y, Kvale PA, Rao AV, Jordan MC, Miller A, Glassroth J, Reichman LB, Wallace JM, Hopewell PC. Pulmonary function tests in HIV-infected patients without AIDS. *Am J Respir Crit Care Med* 1995;**152**:738–745.

18. O'Donnell CR, Bader MB, Zibrak JD, Jensen WA, Rose RM. Abnormal airway function in individuals with the acquired immunodeficiency syndrome. *Chest* 1988;**94**:945–948.

19. Nichols D, Dopico GA, Braun S, Imbeau S, Peters ME, Rankin J. Acute and chronic pulmonary function changes in allergic bronchopulmonary aspergillosis. *Am J Med* 1979;**67**:631–637.

20. Fisher LR, Cawley MID, Holgate ST. Relation between chest expansion, pulmonary function, and exercise tolerance in patients with ankylosing spondylitis. *Ann Rheum Dis* 1990;**49**:921–925.

21. Chilvers ER, Whyte MKB, Jackson JE, Allison DJ, Hughes JMB. Effect of percutaneous transcatheter embolisation on pulmonary function, right-to-left shunt and arterial oxygenation in patients with pulmonary arteriovenous malformations. *Am Rev Respir Dis* 1990;**142**:420–425.

22. Hanson CA, Ritter AB, Duran DJ. Ascites: its effect upon static inflation of the respiratory system. *Am Rev Respir Dis* 1990;**142**:39–42.

23. Lund MB, Kongerud J, Brinch L, Evensen SA, Boe J. Decreased lung function in one year survivors of allogenic bone marrow transplantation conditioned with high-dose busulphan and cyclophosphamide.*Eur Respir J* 1995;**8**:1269–1274.

24. Wright JL, Cagle P, Churg A, Colby TV, Myers J. State of the art: disease of the small airways. *Am Rev Respir Dis* 1992;**146**:240–262.

25. Wagner PD. Impairment of gas exchange in liver cirrhosis. *Eur Respir J* 1995;**8**:1993–1995.

26. Braun SR, Birnbaum ML, Chopra PS. Postoperative pulmonary function abnormalities in coronary artery revascularization surgery. *Chest* 1978;**73**:316–320.

27. Ries AL, Sosa G, Prewitt L, Friedman PJ, Harwood IR. Restricted pulmonary function in cystic fibrosis. *Chest* 1988;**94**:575–579.

28. Sandler M, Bunn AE, Stewart RI. Cross sectional study of pulmonary function in patients with insulin-dependant diabetes mellitus. *Am Rev Respir Dis* 1987;**135**:223–229.

29. Cooper JAD, White DA, Matthay RA. Drug-induced pulmonary disease: cytotoxic drugs. *Am Rev Respir Dis* 1986;**133**:321–340.

30. Allen JN, Davis WB. Eosinophilic lung diseases. *Am J Respir Crit Care Med* 1994;**150**:1423–1438.

31. Durieu J, Wallaert B, Tonnei A-B. Long-term follow-up of pulmonary function in chronic eosinophilic pneumonia. *Eur Respir J* 1997;**10**:286–291.

32. Wright RS, Levine MS, Bellamy PE, Simmons MS, Batra P, Stevenson LW, Walden JA, Laks H, Tashkin DP. Ventilatory and diffusion abnormalities in potential heart transplant recipients. *Chest* 1990;**98**:816–820.

33. Culham EG, Jimenez HAI, King CE. Thoracic kyphosis, rib mobility, and lung volumes in normal women and women with osteoporosis. *Spine* 1994;**19**:1250–1255.

34. Bolliger CT, Jordan P, Soler M, Stulz P, Tamm M, Wyser Ch, Gonon M, Perruchoud AP. Pulmonary function and exercise capacity after lung resection. *Eur Respir J* 1996;**9**:415–421.

35. Braun NMT, Aroroa NS, Rochester DF. Respiratory muscle and pulmonary function in polymyositis and other proximal myopathies. *Thorax* 1983;**38**:616–623.

36: Jenkins SC, Moxham J. The effects of mild obesity on lung function. Resp Med 1991;**85**:309–311.

37. De Bruin PFC, De Bruin VMS, Lees AJ, Pride NB. Effect of treatment on airway dynamics and respiratory muscle strength in Parkinson's disease. *Am Rev Respir Dis* 1993;**148**:1576–1580.

38. DeTroyer A, Desir D, Copinschi G. Regression of lung size in adults with growth hormone deficiency. *Q J Med* 1980;**49**:329–340.

39. Harrison BDW, Millhouse KA, Harrington M, Nabarro JDN. Lung function in acromegaly. *Q J Med* 1978;**47**:517–532.

40. Gilmartin JJ, Wright AJ, Gibson GJ. Effects of pneumothorax or pleural effusion on pulmonary function. *Thorax* 1985;**40**:60–65.

41. Krumholz RA, Echt CR, Ross JC. Pulmonary diffusing capacity, capillary blood volume, lung volumes, and mechanics of ventilation in early and late pregnancy. *J Lab Clin Med* 1964;**63**:648–655.

42. Burke CM, Glanville AR, Morris AJR, Rubin D, Harvey JA, Theodore J, Robin ED. Pulmonary function in advanced pulmonary hypertension. *Thorax* 1987;**42**:131–135.

43. Lipscomb DJ, Patel K, Hughes JMB. Interpretation of increases in the transfer coeficient for carbon monoxide (Tlco/VA or Kco). *Thorax* 1979;**33**:728–733.

44. Mousas B, Raffin TA, Epstein AH, Link CJ. Pulmonary radiation injury. *Chest* 1997;**111**:1061–1078.

45. Moinard J. Guenard H. Membrane diffusion of the lungs in patients with chronic renal failure. *Eur Respir J* 1993;**6**:225–230.

46. Singh S, Dale A, Morgan B, Sahebjami H. Serial studies of pulmonary function in continuous ambulatory peritoneal dialysis. *Chest* 1984;**86**:874–877.

47. Kearon C, Viviani GR, Kikley A, Killian KJ. Factors detemining pulmonary function in adolescent idiopathic thoracic scoliosis. *Am Rev Respir Dis* 1993;**148**:288–294.

48. Miller GJ, Serjeant GR. An assessment of lung volumes and gas transfer in sickle cell anaemia. *Thorax* 1971;**26**:309–315.

49. Bredin CP. Pulmonary function in long-term survivors of thoracoplasty. *Chest* 1989;**95**:18–20.

50. Freedman S. Lung volumes, and distensibility, and maximum respiratory pressures in thyroid disease before and after treatment. *Thorax* 1978;**33**:785–790.

51. Fuleihan FJD, Abboud RT, Balikian JP, Nucho CHN. Pulmonary alveolar microlithiasis: lung function in five cases. *Thorax* 1969;**26**:704–711.

52. Selecky PA, Wasserman K, Benfield JR, Lippman M. The clinical and physiological effect of whole-lung lavage in pulmonary alveolar proteinosis: a ten-year experience. *Ann Thorac Surg* 1977;**24**:451–461.

53. Cordier JF, Loire R, Brune J. Amyloidosis of the lower respiratory tract. *Chest* 1986;**90**:827–831.

54. Hoffman L, Cohn JE, Gaensler EA. Respiratory abnormalities in eosinophilic granuloma of the lung: long term study of five cases. *N Engl J Med* 1962;**267**:577–589.

55. Burger CD Hyatt RE, Staats BA. Pulmonary mechanics in lymphangioleiomyomatosis. *Am Rev Respir Dis* 1991;**143**:1030–1033.

9: SERIAL TESTS

In Chapter 3 we mentioned paired measurements of FEV1 and VC in the context of testing the reversibility of airflow obstruction. Lung volumes and transfer factor are often recorded on several occasions in the same subject, usually to monitor progression of disease and the response to therapy. Let's look at how we assess such a series of results.

TWO SETS OF LUNG FUNCTION TESTS

The following results were obtained in a patient with fibrosing alveolitis. Has there been any significant deterioration over six months?

PATIENT 9.01

Sex:	Female	Height (m):	1.64
Age (yrs):	75	Weight (kg):	90
Tobacco:	Non-smoker	BMI (kg/m²):	33

	19/1/89	19/7/89
Spirometry:		
FEV1 (L)	1.05	0.95
VC (L)	1.40	1.25
FEV1/VC (%)	75	76
Lung Volumes: (Helium dilution)		
RV (L)	1.11	0.95
FRC (L)	1.60	1.39
TLC (L)	2.51	2.20
Gas Transfer: (CO single breath, Hb=13.8 g/dl)		
TLCO (SI)	3.80	3.74
KCO (SI)	1.58	1.76

A common figure used for the repeatability of lung function tests is 10%. However, 10% of an FEV1 of 5 L is 500mls, whereas 10% of an FEV1 of 0.5 L is only 50mls, as we noted in Chapter 3. In fact, we know that for FEV1 a repeat test is likely to be within 0.2 L of the initial value, irrespective of what the intital value is[1]. The corresponding figure for VC is 0.35 L. (You can calculate that 0.2 L is 40% of an FEV1 of 0.5 L and 4% of 5 L, so it's clearly much easier for a patient with small lungs to reach the 10% threshold.) Similar reproducability data are not available for other lung volumes or transfer factor, so we are stuck with 10%. Let's express the changes in our patient in this way:

PATIENT 9.01

Sex:	Female	Height (m):	1.64
Age (yrs):	75	Weight (kg):	90
Tobacco:	Non-smoker	BMI (kg/m²):	33

	19/1/89	19/7/89	*Change* (%)
Spirometry:			
FEV1 (L)	1.05	0.95	-9
VC (L)	1.40	1.25	-11
FEV1/VC (%)	75	76	+1
Lung Volumes: (Helium dilution)			
RV (L)	1.11	0.95	-14
FRC (L)	1.60	1.39	-13
TLC (L)	2.51	2.20	-12
Gas Transfer: (CO single breath, Hb=13.8 g/dl)			
TLCO (SI)	3.80	3.74	-2
KCO (SI)	1.58	1.76	+11

By "Change" I mean (Test2 - Test1)/Test1, expressed as a percentage. In the spirometry results the VC has fallen by 11%, but we know that changes in VC of less than 0.35 L are less than the reproducability of the test. The changes in lung volumes are greater than 10%, but nevertheless pretty small. TLCO has hardly changed, so we can safely say *"No significant change"*.

We can get over the problem of 10% representing a very small change when the intial value is itself very low by using 10% of the predicted value, rather than 10% of the first test, i.e. (Test2 - Test1)/Predicted.

PATIENT 9.01

Sex	Female	Height (m)	1.64
Age (yrs)	75	Weight (kg)	90
Tobacco	Non-smoker	BMI (kg/m²)	19

	Predicted	*19/1/89*	*19/7/89*	*Change (% pred)*
Spirometry:				
FEV1 (L)	2.00	1.05	0.95	-5
VC (L)	2.43	1.40	1.25	-6
FEV1/VC (%)	75	75	76	+1
Lung Volumes: (Helium dilution)				
RV (L)	2.17	1.11	0.95	-7
FRC (L)	2.75	1.60	1.39	-8
TLC (L)	5.03	2.51	2.20	-6
Gas Transfer: (CO single breath, Hb=13.8 g/dl)				
TLCO (SI)	7.00	3.80	3.74	-1
KCO (SI)	1.55	1.58	1.76	+12

Now all the changes (except KCO) are less than 10%. This approach is now accepted for spirometry, as we have seen in Chapter 3, but curiously it is little used for other lung function tests.

MULTIPLE SETS OF LUNG FUNCTION TESTS

In the previous example, we dismissed a change of 150mls in VC as insignificant. If on the next occassion the test were performed VC was another 150mls lower, we would be much more suspicious that there had been a deterioration. Let's look at these VC results in the series of results from which they were taken:

PATIENT 9.01

	1/89	*7/89*	*1/90*	*1/91*	*9/91*
Spirometry:					
VC (L)	1.40	1.25	1.20	1.10	1.05

Each successive result shows a decline, so clearly this signifies deteriorating lung function (which is greater than normal ageing - see later in this chapter). We could perform statistical analysis to tell us whether there was any significant change with time, or even produce a prediction of the next result, together with confidence intervals. (When plotting the data, we could also use mathematical techniques to smooth the data.) In clinical practice this sort of sophisticated analysis is seldom, if ever, carried out.

PRESENTATION OF RESULTS

When measurements of lung volumes and gas transfer have been measured on several occasions, presentation of the results in the form of a table can be pretty indigestible. Here is the full series in the patient we have been looking at so far:

PATIENT 9.01

	1/87	6/87	9/87	3/88	9/88	1/89	7/89	1/90	1/91	9/91
Spirometry:										
FEV1 (L)	1.15	1.20	1.15	1.15	1.11	1.05	0.95	0.95	0.85	0.80
VC (L)	1.35	1.50	1.40	1.35	1.35	1.40	1.25	1.20	1.10	1.05
FEV1/VC	85	80	82	85	82	75	76	76	77	76
Lung Volumes: (Helium dilution)										
RV (L)	1.58	1.46	1.32	1.08	1.15	1.11	0.95	1.05	1.00	0.96
FRC (L)	1.91	1.79	1.75	1.52	1.59	1.60	1.39	1.49	1.45	1.44
TLC (L)	2.93	2.96	2.72	2.43	2.50	2.51	2.20	2.25	2.10	2.01
Gas Transfer: (CO single breath, Hb=13.8 g/dl)										
TLCO (SI)	5.67	5.30	3.93	4.52	4.22	3.74	3.68	3.63	3.46	3.16
KCO(SI)	1.98	1.86	1.54	1.81	1.73	1.58	1.76	1.64	1.64	1.67

The pair of results we considered in isolation earlier, 1/89 and 7/89, can now be seen in context. In fact, giving all the lung volumes in this instance is unnecessary, as you can see if we plot them as a percentage of the starting value:

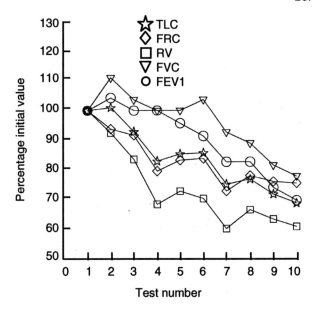

Figure 9.1

They all change in the same direction, not surprisingly. It would be a lot easier to see a trend if we just look at one volume, such as VC, though FEV1 or TLC (or even VA) would also be good candidates. We will still need TLCO as an index of gas transfer, but since VA is likely also to parallel changes in other lung volumes, KCO will be unnecessary. (In fibrosing alveolitis, VC or TLC are the most important predictors of progression[2], with TLCO adding surprisingly little. TLCO can still be useful during therapeutic trials).

Time for the old template again, to blank out the redundant information:

PATIENT 9.02

	1/87	6/87	9/87	3/88	9/88	1/89	7/89	1/90	1/91	9/91
Spirometry:										
FEV1 (L)										
VC (L)	1.35	1.50	1.40	1.35	1.35	1.40	1.25	1.20	1.10	1.05
FEV1/VC										
Lung Volumes: (Helium dilution)										
RV (L)										
FRC (L)										
TLC (L)										
Gas Transfer: (CO single breath, Hb=13.8 g/dl)										
TLCO (SI)	5.67	5.30	3.93	4.52	4.22	3.74	3.68	3.63	3.46	3.16
KCO (SI)										

A graphical plot of these two parameters is even easier to spot trends on, for example in the following series of tests from a patient with systemic sclerosis:

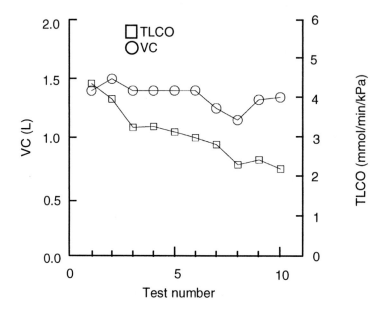

Figure 9.2

PERCENT PREDICTED AND STANDARDISED RESIDUALS

We have spent much of this book comparing lung function test results to the predicted values, using either standardised residuals or percentages. The prediction equations in common usage are all from cross-sectional studies, and cannot be used for longitudinal comparisons. Do not look at the SRs or percent predicted values when comparing two or more sets of test results.

In the prediction equation for FVC in males, the factor (- 0.026 x age) is used, predicted FVC being in litres and age in years. This implies a linear decline in FVC in normal adult males of 26mls/year. In fact, FVC is fairly stable until the age of around 40 years, after which there is a decline, the rate of which accelerates to about 50mls/year by 60 years of age[3]. (Most of this change is attributable to an increase in RV.) Unfortunately, there are very few satisfactory longitudinal studies reported, and they are almost entirely confined to spirometry.

SUMMARY

☞ To be significant, any change in a lung function test measured on two occasions should be larger than the reproducibility of the test, and greater than 10% of the predicted value for that test in that individual.

☞ Longitudinal changes in lung function are often best identified by looking at a limited number of test parameters, preferably in graphical presentation.

☞ Percent predicted and standardised residuals should not be used in the assessment of longitudinal changes in lung function.

REFERENCES

1. Van Pelt W, Borsboom GJJM, Rijcken B, Schouten JP, Van Zomeren BC, Quanjer PH. Discrepancies between longitudinal and cross-sectional change in ventilatory function in 12 years of follow-up. *Am J Respir Crit Med* 1994;**149**:1218–1226.

2. Erbes R, Schaberg T, Loddenkemper R. Lung function tests in patients with idiopathic pulmonary fibrosis. Are they helpful for predicting outcome? *Chest* 1997;**111**:51–57.

3. Tweedale PM, Alexander F, McHardy GJR. Short term variability in FEV1 and bronchodilator responsiveness in patients with obstructive ventilatory defects. *Thorax* 1987;**42**:487–490.

10: BLOOD GASES

There are two main aspects to a set of arterial blood gas results, gas exchange and acid-base balance, although obviously the two are closely linked. In a book on lung function, it makes sense to look at gas exchange first. (I shall assume that the sample has been taken correctly and analysed promptly - on a machine that has been maintained and calibrated correctly.)

GAS EXCHANGE - PaO$_2$

The first question we must ask ourselves when looking at some blood gas results is "Is the patient hypoxic?". (By hypoxic I really mean hypoxaemic). The following result was obtained from a patient presenting to the Accident and Emergency Department with asthma:

PATIENT 10.01

	Measured	Normal Range
Blood gases:		
PaO$_2$ (kPa)	13.4	12.0 - 15.0
(mmHg)	100	90 - 112

(The use of SI units for arterial gases is far from universal, so I've given the results in mmHg alongside.)

Although it would be logical to use standardised residuals to delineate normal from abnormal for blood gases, just as we have done for other lung function results, the use of SRs is as yet almost unheard of in this context so I've stuck to normal ranges. These are for arterial samples; PaO$_2$ is slightly lower if the arterialized capillary technique is used[1].

Returning to our example, as you can see these results are normal. However, it is impossible to interpret PaO$_2$ without knowing what the inspired oxygen concentration was. Air contains approximately 21% oxygen, sometimes expressed as a Fraction of the inspired gas, abbreviated as FiO$_2$. (Strictly speaking, the FiO$_2$ for a patient breathing air is 0.21 rather than 21%, but since most oxygen masks refer to percentages I have used these in preference to fractions.) If Patient 10.01 was breathing 60% oxygen at the time the sample was taken, a PaO$_2$ of 13.4 would indicate a problem with gas exchange.

The next sample was taken from a patient with left lower lobe pneumonia:

PATIENT 10.02

FiO$_2$: 40%	Measured	Normal Range
Blood gases:		
PaO$_2$ (kPa)	12.5	12.0 - 15.0
(mmHg)	94	90 - 112

The PaO$_2$ is normal, but obviously much less than it should be for someone breathing such a high concentration of oxygen. How much less? It is possible to calculate what the PaO$_2$ should be for a normal subject breathing 40% oxygen. This involves estimation of the alveolar oxygen concentration using the alveolar air equation, which most of us have to look up every time we need to use it. Then you subtract the normal alveolar-arterial difference, which unfortunately varies with FiO$_2$, so you would need to look that up as well. (FiO$_2$/PaO$_2$ has been advocated as an index which is easier to calculate and less dependant on FiO$_2$, but it is not widely used).

These calculations are of dubious relevance in clinical practice, where the FiO$_2$ is estimated from the label on the mask rather than actually measured. As a rough rule of thumb, if the PaCO$_2$ is normal the PaO$_2$ for different FiO$_2$s can be estimated as follows:

PaO$_2$ (kPa) = FiO$_2$ (%) x 0.75
or
PaO$_2$ (mmHg) = FiO$_2$ (%) x 5

Our first question needs a qualification - "Is the patient hypoxic, or would they be if they were breathing air ?" Looking back to Patient 10.02 on 40% oxygen, our rough rule of thumb suggests that the PaO$_2$ should be about 30 kPa (40 x 0.75) or 200 mmHg (40 x 5) so we could say "*PaO$_2$ not as high as expected for inspired oxygen concentration*".

Hypoxia can be caused by several different factors - hypoventilation, impaired diffusion, ventilation/perfusion imbalance and shunts. It is not usually possible to tell from the blood gas results which of these is responsible for the low PaO$_2$, although the PaCO$_2$ may give some clues, as we shall see shortly.

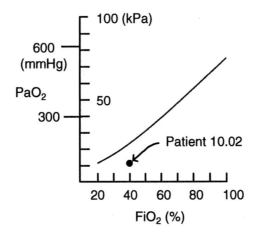

Figure 10.1

GAS EXCHANGE - PaCO$_2$

Hypoxia usually stimulates the patient to increase ventilation. PaCO$_2$ invariably falls as alveolar ventilation rises. The next patient was suspected of having had a pulmonary embolus:

PATIENT 10.03

FiO$_2$: 21%		
	Measured	*Normal Range*
Blood gases:		
PaO$_2$ (kPa)	9.6	12.0 - 15.0
(mmHg)	72	90 - 112
PaCO$_2$ (kPa)	2.9	4.5 - 6.1
(mmHg)	22	34 - 46

These results show that the patient is hypoxic, which has stimulated ventilation and therefore lowered the PaCO$_2$. Note that we are talking about alveolar ventilation rather than total ventilation - arterial gas results by themselves cannot tell us anything about dead space ventilation. We can conclude *"Mild hypoxia with compensatory hyperventilation"*.

When PaCO$_2$ is low, there is more room for oxygen in the alveolar gas. Hyperventilation in normal subjects leads to a PaO$_2$ at, or just above, the upper end of the normal range, as in this anxious patient with chest pain:

PATIENT 10.04

FiO_2: 21%	Measured	Normal Range
Blood gases:		
PaO_2 (kPa)	16.1	12.0 - 15.0
(mmHg)	121	90 - 112
$PaCO_2$ (kPa)	1.3	4.5 - 6.1
(mmHg)	10	34 - 46

Time for another rule of thumb: if the patient is breathing air, the sum of the PaO_2 and $PaCO_2$ should be around 17 kPa (130 mmHg) if the lungs are normal. This is the case in Patient 10.03, who is probably hyperventilating in response to the pain. (Since it is difficult to get your $PaCO_2$ below 1 kPa (7.5 mmHg), it follows that the highest PaO_2 should be about 16 kPa (120 mmHg) - values above this indicate that the patient must have been receiving supplementary oxygen.) If we look back to the previous patient, we can see that the PaO_2 is not as high as it should be if the lungs were normal.

The 17 kPa (130 mmHg) rule applies to hypoventilation as much as hyperventilation. The next patient had poliomyelitis as a teenager, and had become more tired over a number of years:

PATIENT 10.05

FiO_2: 21%	Measured	Normal Range
Blood gases:		
PaO_2 (kPa)	4.0	12.0 - 15.0
(mmHg)	30	90 - 112
$PaCO_2$ (kPa)	12.1	4.5 - 6.1
(mmHg)	91	34 - 46

The high $PaCO_2$ means that alveolar ventilation is low, but the sum of $PaCO_2$ and PaO_2 is 16.1. We could conclude *"The elevation of $PaCO_2$ indicates alveolar hypoventilation, which is probably of sufficient severity to explain the hypoxia."*

Hypercapnia with reciprocal and appropriate change in PaO_2 is unusual - it is much more common for alveolar ventilation and gas exchange both to be abnormal, as in this patient with COAD:

PATIENT 10.06

FiO$_2$: 21%		
	Measured	*Normal Range*
Blood gases:		
PaO$_2$ (kPa)	5.4	12.0 - 15.0
(mmHg)	41	90 - 112
PaCO$_2$ (kPa)	7.1	4.5 - 6.1
(mmHg)	54	34 - 46

The high PaCO$_2$ means that alveolar ventilation is low, (although total ventilation may be high). If this were pure hypoventilation we would expect a PaO$_2$ of 10 kPa, so there must be impaired oxygenation. This leads us to *"Hypercapnia indicating alveolar hypoventilation, but very low PaO$_2$ indicates an additional gas exchange problem"*. Acid base balance will give us a clue as to whether this is an acute or chronic problem.

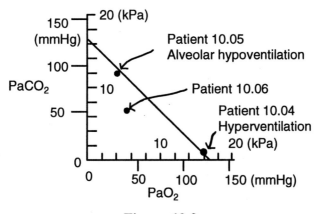

Figure 10.2

RESPIRATORY ACIDOSIS

Acid base balance is much less complicated than it often seems. Part of the confusion which surrounds the topic comes from the use of base excess, total CO$_2$, standard bicarbonate, etc. In almost all cases, the actual bicarbonate level is all that we need. The second factor which muddies the water is the use of examples which, although they illustrate the biochemistry and physiology well, are extremely rare in clinical practice. There aren't that many patients around who have had their ureters implanted into their colon, overdose on bicarbonate of soda and then have an acute hypercapnic exacerbation of their chronic bronchitis. In most instances we have some clinical information anyway, and we don't have to try and work backwards from the blood gas results.

Alveolar hypoventilation leads to a high $PaCO_2$. When this occurs acutely, the result is an acidosis:

PATIENT 10.07

FiO$_2$: 35%	Measured	Normal Range
Blood gases:		
PaO$_2$ (kPa)	12.4	12.0 - 15.0
(mmHg)	93	90 - 112
PaCO$_2$ (kPa)	11.4	4.5 - 6.1
(mmHg)	86	34 - 46
pH	7.15	7.35 - 7.45
H+ (nmol/L)	71	35 - 45
HCO$_3$ (mmol/L)	29	22 - 29

If we stick to our routine of looking first at PaO_2, we see that this is within the normal range, but not as high as we would expect on 35% oxygen. The elevation of $PaCO_2$ tells us that the alveoli are inadequately ventilated. An acidosis is present, and our first thought is that this is related to the elevated $PaCO_2$, in other words a respiratory acidosis. (In a non-respiratory or "metabolic" acidosis the bicarbonate level is low, as we shall see shortly.) The fact that in this patient the bicarbonate is normal confirms that this is a respiratory problem, and that compensatory mechanisms have not yet come into play. We interpret this as *"There is an acute respiratory acidosis, with a PaO$_2$ lower than would be expected for the FiO$_2$."* We can only speculate as to the cause of the impaired oxygenation, and our 17 kPa rule of thumb cannot help us since the patient is breathing supplemental oxygen.

$PaCO_2$ is often plotted against pH (or H+) to show the differences between various acid base disturbances. In the case of an acute respiratory acidosis, the patient moves into the upper right-hand quadrant of the plot where pH is low and $PaCO_2$ is high:

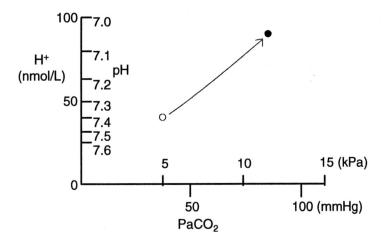

Figure 10.3

Bicarbonate "isopleths" can be added to this graph, in our example the patient moving along one:

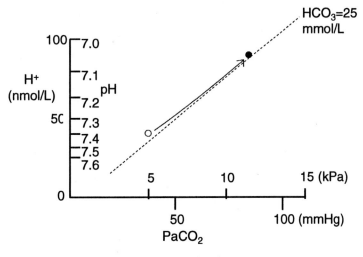

Figure 10.4

If the $PaCO_2$ remains elevated for more than a few hours, the bicarbonate level rises in an attempt by the kidneys to restore the pH to normal:

PATIENT 10.08

FiO$_2$: 21%	Measured	Normal Range
PaO$_2$ (kPa)	4.8	12.0 - 15.0
(mmHg)	36	90 -112
PaCO$_2$ (kPa)	8.1	4.5 - 6.1
(mmHg)	61	34 - 46
pH	7.35	7.35 - 7.45
H+ (nmol/L)	45	35 - 45
HCO$_3$ (mmol/L)	33	22 - 29

This shows that a respiratory acidosis has been compensated for, restoring the pH to within the normal range. We can say *"Chronic hypercapnic respiratory failure"*. Compensation is often incomplete, restoring pH towards or just into the normal range.

On our PaCO$_2$/pH plot, the patient moves downwards from the acute respiratory acidosis position. The relationship between this shift and changes in bicarbonate is demonstrated by the change to an isopleth which represents a higher bicarbonate concentration:

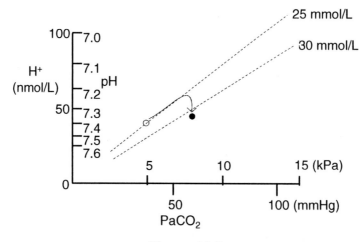

Figure 10.5

RESPIRATORY ALKALOSIS

If hyperventilation leads to an acute fall in $PaCO_2$, the pH rises:

PATIENT 10.09

FiO$_2$: 21%	Measured	Normal Range
Blood gases:		
PaO$_2$ (kPa)	9.6	12.0 - 15.0
(mmHg)	73	90 - 112
PaCO$_2$ (kPa)	2.9	4.5 - 6.1
(mmHg)	22	34 - 46
pH	7.56	7.35 - 7.45
H+ (nmol/L)	28	35 - 45
HCO$_3$ (mmol/L)	22	22 - 29

The cause of the hyperventilation is indicated by the fact that the PaO_2 is low: *"Hypoxia with compensatory hyperventilation and acute respiratory alkalosis"*.

Again, if the $PaCO_2$ remains low for more than a few hours, renal compensation comes into play. In the case of a respiratory alkalosis, the bicarbonate level falls:

PATIENT 10.10

FiO$_2$: 21%	Measured	Normal Range
Blood gases:		
PaO$_2$ (kPa)	17.9	12.0 - 15.0
(mmHg)	134	90 - 112
PaCO$_2$ (kPa)	2.6	4.5 - 6.1
(mmHg)	20	34 - 46
pH	7.49	7.35 - 7.45
H+ (nmol/L)	32	35 - 45
HCO$_3$ (mmol/L)	15	22 - 29

We can therefore conclude *"Chronic respiratory alkalosis"*.

METABOLIC ACIDOSIS

If an acidosis is non-respiratory or "metabolic" in origin, then the pH and bicarbonate will be low. The low pH is a potent stimulus to respiration, so the $PaCO_2$ is usually low. This respiratory response is very rapid (unlike the metabolic compensation for a primary respiratory disturbance) and it is unusual to see a metabolic acidosis without a low $PaCO_2$ (unless the patient is unable to produce a ventilatory response). Patient 10.11 was known to be diabetic and was admitted with vomiting:

PATIENT 10.11

	Measured	Normal Range
FiO_2: 28%		
Blood gases:		
PaO_2 (kPa)	19.0	12.0 - 15.0
(mmHg)	139	90 - 112
$PaCO_2$ (kPa)	1.4	4.5 - 6.1
(mmHg)	10	34 - 46
pH	6.90	7.35 - 7.45
H+ (nmol/L)	126	35 - 45
HCO_3 (mmol/L)	2	22 - 29

Working down the results, the PaO_2 is probably fine for 28% oxygen, but the $PaCO_2$ is low. The pH and bicarbonate indicate a non-respiratory acidosis, so the low $PaCO_2$ is a secondary phenomenum.

METABOLIC AND RESPIRATORY ACIDOSIS

Patients with acute hypercapnic respiratory failure are often very unwell, with hypotension and poor peripheral perfusion. Arterial oxygen saturation is low anyway, and so it is not surprising that if tissues have a poor blood flow they will have to metabolise anaerobically, leading to production of lactate. The respiratory and metabolic acidosis both lower the pH, the $PaCO_2$ is high from the alveolar hyoventilation and the bicarbonate is low from the non-respiratory acidosis:

PATIENT 10.12

FiO$_2$: 100%	Measured	Normal Range
Blood gases:		
PaO$_2$ (kPa)	7.1	12.0 - 15.0
(mmHg)	53	90 - 112
PaCO$_2$ (kPa)	15.7	4.5 - 6.1
(mmHg)	118	34 - 46
pH	6.8	7.35 - 7.45
H+ (nmol/L)	158	35 - 45
HCO$_3$ (mmol/L)	18	22 - 29

The high PaCO$_2$ would be associated with a normal or high bicarbonate if this were purely respiratory. On the other hand, if the acidosis were entirely non-respiratory, the PaCO$_2$ should be low.

OTHER DISORDERS OF ACID-BASE BALANCE

The slant I have taken to this topic has been unashamedly "respiratory". There are other facets to acid-base balance, but I don't propose to give any more examples. The main disturbance we have not considered is metabolic alkalosis, which is much rarer than those we have discussed thus far. It can be seen in combination with a respiratory acidosis or alkalosis, but I think we run the risk of confusing the picture by considering these rarities further.

SUMMARY

☞ PaO_2 values can only be interpreted properly if we know the FiO_2.

☞ In a patient with normal lungs, the sum of PaO_2 and $PaCO_2$ should be approximately 17 kPa (or 130 mmHg) if they are breathing air.

☞ In respiratory acidosis, the bicarbonate level is normal acutely but elevated if hypercapnia is sustained for more than a few hours.

☞ In respiratory alkalosis, the bicarbonate level falls if alveolar hyperventilation is sustained for more than a few hours.

☞ A metabolic acidosis, with a low bicarbonate, stimulates respiration and causes a low $PaCO_2$.

☞ In an acidosis, if the bicarbonate is low and the $PaCO_2$ is high, the acidosis is of mixed respiratory and non-respiratory origin.

REFERENCES

1. Sauty A, Uldry C, Debetaz L-F, Leuenberger P, Fitting J-W. Differences in PO_2 and PCO_2 between arterial and arterialized earlobe samples. *Eur Respir J* 1996;**9**:186–189.

11: TESTS OF RESPIRATORY MUSCLE FUNCTION

We noted the effects of respiratory muscle weakness on flow-volume loops and lung volumes in previous chapters, but specific tests of respiratory muscle function are becoming routine in many lung function laboratories. I do not propose to devote space to the more invasive techniques such as measurement of transdiaphragmatic pressure and phrenic nerve conduction time, but some of the simpler tests merit consideration. Before we consider these, let's double back for a moment to spirometry and look at the effect of posture.

POSTURAL CHANGES IN VC

When we are in the upright position, either seated or standing, the contents of the abdominal cavity are pulled down by the force of gravity. On changing to the supine position, this gravitational force is eliminated, and were it not for active contraction of the diaphragm, the abdominal contents would ascend into the thorax. If the diaphragm is paralysed, this is exactly what happens, and the patient becomes breathless.

In a normal subject, any fall in VC between the upright and supine positions is minimal, normally less than 15%. Quite dramatic differences can be seen in patients with bilateral diaphragm paralysis:

PATIENT 11.01

Sex:	Male	Height (m):	1.68
Age (yrs):	72	Weight (kg):	90
Tobacco:	Non-smoker	BMI (kg/m²):	32

	Measured
Vital Capacity:	
Seated (L)	2.83
Supine (L)	1.60
Seated-supine (L)	1.23
(% seated)	43

Clearly there is a marked fall in VC when the patient lies down, so we could infer *"Marked fall in VC in the supine posture, consistent with the bilateral diaphragm weakness"*. The changes in unilateral paralysis are much less, in the order of 15-30%[1].

Although 15% is the cut-off for subjects with fairly normal lungs, much greater falls can be seen in patients with abnormal lungs who do not have any suggestion of diaphragmatc weakness. It is important, therefore, to look at the conventional spirometry results first:

PATIENT 11.02

Sex:	Female	Height (m):	1.70	
Age (yrs):	60	Weight (kg):	78	
Tobacco:	Smoker	BMI (kg/m²):	29	

	Measured	*Predicted*	*% Pred*	*SR*
Spirometry:				
FEV1 (L)	1.19		45	-3.8
VC (L)	2.41		78	-1.6
FEV1/VC (%)	49		63	-4.4
VC supine (L)	1.85			
Seated-supine	0.56			
(% seated)	23	<15		

This fall in VC must be interpreted with caution in view of the severity of airflow obstruction. Such patients can show falls in VC of up to 40% in the absence of any evidence of diaphragm paralysis, as can patients with restrictive lung problems[2]. *"Obstructive spirometry. The fall in VC in the supine posture is normal for a patient with airflow obstruction of this severity"*.

MAXIMUM MOUTH PRESSURES

The most commonly used tests of respiratory muscle strength are maximum mouth pressures, whereby the patient makes a maximum inspiratory or expiratory manoeuvre against an occluded mouthpiece. A small leak is made in the mouthpiece in order to minimise the contribution of buccal muscles, and during expiratory efforts the patient should press with their hands against their cheeks for the same reason. The results are most commonly expressed in cmH$_2$O, or sometimes mmHg. (The appropriate SI unit is kPa.)

RV, TLC OR FRC ?

If you want to generate the highest expiratory pressure you can, you take a deep breath in before blowing into the mouth pressure meter. However, at TLC the pressure you record will include the inward elastic recoil pressure of your lungs and chest wall, as well as that generated by your expiratory muscles. If you were at FRC you would record a lower pressure, but at least we would know that it was all muscle. (Similar arguments apply to the use of RV or FRC for maximum inspiratory pressure.) The normal ranges differ depending upon which volume is used, but this effect is surprisingly small[3].

TECHNIQUE

When we considered spirometry, we noted that inspecting the volume-time trace enabled us to assess how well the patient had performed the manoeuvre. Sometimes we might say *"VC of 1.6 L is likely to be an underestimate in view of poor test technique"*. VC may be underestimated, but not overestimated. MIP and MEP may be underestimated if the patient does not suck or blow hard enough, or if there are leaks around the mouthpiece. They may also be overestimated if the subject uses their buccal muscles. This latter problem can be minimised by incorporating a small leak in the mouthpiece, asking the patient to support their cheeks with their hands during the manoeuvre, and taking the maximum pressure that can be sustained for one second. Whenever possible, look at the raw data before coming to any conclusions.

When the test has been performed well, a plateau of pressure will be seen:

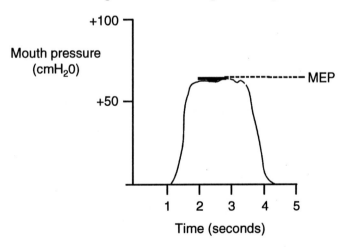

Figure 11.1

Poor technique is associated with a poorly sustained maximum pressure, and the one second average is clearly not a good representation of expiratory muscle strength:

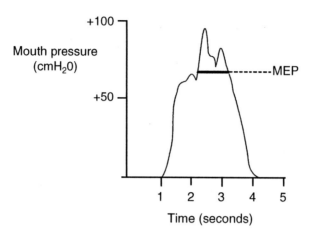

Figure 11.2

NORMAL RANGE

Compared to the equations for lung volumes and transfer factor, predicted values for MIP and MEP are based on much smaller numbers of subjects. Quality control over the technical aspects of recording mouth pressures is also still fairly rudimentary. For the present, the best we can do is choose one of the larger normal range studies which used a population which is likely to be similar to that from which our patients come, and then take care that the technique used in our laboratory to record the pressures is a close as possible to that in the study we are going to use as a reference.

One of the largest studies of MIP and MEP[4] gives the following means and standard deviations:

	Males	Females
MIP (cmH$_2$O)	118 (37)	84 (30)
MEP (cmH$_2$O)	134 (31)	89 (21)

The standard deviations are pretty large, and if we use +/- (1.64 x RSD) to define the normal range, the lower limits are as follows:

	Males	Females
MIP (cmH$_2$O)	> 57	> 35
MEP (cmH$_2$O)	> 83	> 55

In this and other studies, normal values have been influenced to a minor extent by height, weight and age. However, these effects are small compared to the reproducability of the technique, and can probably be ignored in clinical practice when mouth pressures are used as a screening method for respiratory muscle weakness. Values greater than the normal range are of no clinical relevance, so all we need to do is compare the measured value to the lower limit of normal.

Let's look again at Patient 11.01, with suspected diaphragm weakness:

PATIENT 11.01

Sex:	Male	Height (m):	1.68
Age (yrs):	72	Weight (kg):	90
Tobacco:	Non-smoker	BMI (kg/m²):	32

	Measured	Predicted
Vital Capacity:		
Seated (L)	2.83	
Supine (L)	1.60	
Seated-supine	1.23	
(% seated)	43	< 15
Maximum Mouth Pressures:		
MIP (cmH2O)	44	> 57
MEP (cmH2O)	128	> 83

As we might expect, inspiratory pressures are low, consistent with our initial impression that the diaphragm was weak. Expiratory muscle strength is well preserved.

As with postural changes in VC, MIP and MEP are difficult to interpret in a patient with abnormal lungs:

PATIENT 11.02

Sex:	Female	Height (m):	1.70
Age (yrs):	60	Weight (kg):	78
Tobacco:	Smoker	BMI (kg/m²):	27

	Measured	Predicted	% Pred	SR
Spirometry:				
FEV1 (L)	1.19		45	-3.8
VC (L)	2.41		78	-1.6
FEV1/VC (%)	49		63	-4.4
VC supine (L)	1.85			
Seated-supine	0.56			
(% seated)	23	< 15		
Maximum Mouth Pressures:				
MIP (cmH$_2$O)	28	> 35		
MEP (cmH$_2$O)	74	> 55		

Remember to look at the raw pressure-time trace first to check that MIP was recorded satisfactorily. Even then, we must interpret this minor degree of weakness with caution. An increase in the lung volume at which the MIP manoeuvre is performed will tend to decrease the pressure generated. This is likely to be the case with airflow obstruction. *"Low MIP and postural fall in VC probably normal for this severity of airflow obstruction, without superimposed muscle weakness"* would be a reasonable interpretation.

NASAL PRESSURES

Static maximal inspiratory and expiratory manoeuvres require a fair amount of practice to yield consistent values in a subject. Sniffing comes to most of us more naturally, and this manoeuvre has been used for many years to assess diahragmatic motion under x-ray screening. Trans-diaphragmatic pressure during sniffs is a useful test of inspiratory muscle function, for which the subject must swallow a pair of balloons or a catheter on which two or more pressure transducers are mounted. The pressure in the upper airway gives an approximation of what is happening to pleural pressure during sniffs, and can be used as a screening test for inspiratory muscle weakness. The best way of doing this to be described to date involves occluding one nostril and sniffing through the other[5]. The pressure is recorded by a pressure transducer in the occluded nostril.

The prediction equations for <u>S</u>niff <u>N</u>asal <u>I</u>nspiratory <u>P</u>ressure (SNIP) using this technique are as follows:

Males: SNIP = 126.8 - (0.42 x Age), RSD 23.8

Females: SNIP = 94.9 - (0.22 x Age), RSD 17.1

Using (1.64 x RSD) to define the normal range, the lower limits of normal can be calculated for each patient:

PATIENT 11.03

Sex:	Female	Height (m):	1.50
Age (yrs):	32	Weight (kg):	60
Tobacco:	Non-smoker	BMI (kg/m²):	27

	Measured	*Predicted*
Maximum Mouth Pressures:		
MIP (cmH$_2$O)	20	> 35
MEP (cmH$_2$O)	25	> 55
SNIP (cmH$_2$O)	31	> 60

Here the low SNIP confirms inspiratory muscle weakness.

SUMMARY

☞ In a normal subject, VC should fall by less than 15% on changing from the upright to supine posture.

☞ In patients with abnormal lungs, postural falls in VC of up to 40% may be seen in the absence of diaphragm paralysis.

☞ Maximum mouth pressure values should be interpreted together with the pressure-time trace recorded during the manoeuvre.

☞ Sniff Nasal Inspiratory Pressure (SNIP) is a useful screening test for inspiratory muscle weakness.

REFERENCES

1. Lisboa C, Pare DD, Pertuze J, Contreras G, Moreno R, Guillemi S, Cruz E. Inspiratory muscle function in unilateral diaphragm paralysis. *Am Rev Respir Dis* 1986;**134**:488–492.

2. Allen SM, Hunt B, Green M. Fall in vital capacity with posture. *Br J Dis Chest* 1985;**79**:267–271.

3. Bruschi C, Cerveri I, Zoia MC, Fanfulla F, Fiorentini M, Casali L, Grassi M, Grassi C. Reference values of maximal respiratory mouth pressures: a population-based study. *Am Rev Respir Dis* 1992;**146**:790–793.

4. Enright PL, Adams AB, Boyle PJR, Sherrill DL. Spirometry and maximal respiratory pressure references from healthy Minnesota 65- to 85-year-old women and men. *Chest* 1995; **108**:663–669.

5. Uldry C, Fitting J-W. Maximal values of sniff nasal inspiratory pressure in healthy subjects. *Thorax* 1995;**50**:371–375.

12: EXERCISE TESTS

Several excellent texts are available on the topic of cardio-respiratory exercise testings (See Bibliography), and if you are regularly involved in reporting exercise tests you will undoubtedly wish to read them. I thought that it would nevertheless be worthwhile to give an overview of the topic, with some guidelines on interpretation.

WHICH PATIENTS?

In the assessment of breathlessness or impaired exercise tolerance, a cardio-respiratory exercise test is usually only carried out after more simple tests have been performed. These tests will usually include measurement of lung volumes, transfer factor, haemoglobin and arterial blood gases. An ECG must be recorded before exercising the patent, and if this is abnormal or if there are any clinical pointers to impaired ventricular function then an echocardiogram may be indicated. Serial peak flow monitoring or a ventilation-perfusion scan may also be performed beforehand, depending upon the clinical circumstances.

These preliminary investigations may all be normal, but we are left with a symptomatic patient. An exercise test may then reveal an abnormality which was not detected by tests performed at rest, and the pattern of abnormality can give us some clues as to the underlying disease process. Alternatively, the exercise test may be normal, in which case many diseases can be excluded as the cause of the patient's symptoms. Characteristic patterns may then point to "psychogenic" or "behavioural" dyspnoea.

We may already know that a patient has respiratory disease, for example, chronic obstructive airways disease, but be puzzled by why they are so symptomatic from what appears to be relatively mild disease. An exercise test enables us to assess the degree of impairment and see if indeed it is the disease which is limiting exercise tolerance. It may reveal other contributing factors, such as poor effort or unfitness, or even unsuspected cardiac disease.

Serial exercise tests can be used to evaluate an intervention, such as drug therapy, surgery, a rehabilitation program, etc.

WHICH TEST?

There are several simple exercise tests, perhaps the most familiar of which is the six minute corridor walk. This is easy to perform and gives an idea of the extent of exercise intolerance but not its cause. The most common reason for exercise testing is to diagnose myocardial ischaemia in a patient with chest pain. By far the majority of such tests are done without analysis of respiratory parameters, and I shall not discuss such "cardiac" tests further.

Steady state exercise tests are beloved of exercise physiologists and are the best way of assessing change after an intervention. However, if you are starting to learn how to interpret exercise tests, you are likely to be looking at data recorded by a computerised system, and the chances are that this will have generated "breath-by-breath" data using a protocol which involves a progressive increase in workload until the patient can go no further. I am going to confine this chapter to the discussion of these tests.

Pulse oximeters are now commonplace in most hospitals, and I shall assume that SaO_2 is measured during the exercise test. Arterial sampling greatly enhances the information which can be obtained from an exercise test, enabling the calculation of alveolar-arterial differences, physiological dead space, etc. However, this practice is far from routine and in the interest of simplicity I shall leave this topic to specialist books on exercise.

PRESENTATION OF EXERCISE DATA

Computers are invaluable for the number crunching aspects of exercise testing, but as we have seen with some other lung function tests, there is a great temptation to use them to derive dozens of different parameters. Moreover, these can be printed out breath-by-breath and plotted against each other ad infinitum. The result is an indigestible booklet, which it is daunting for the uninitiated to even begin to look at. There are a number of key parameters which we need to examine, and thereafter we need to glance at one or two graphs. Ignore all the rest or, even better, stop your computer from printing them out.

MAXIMUM EXERCISE PERFORMANCE

Oxygen uptake

The most important value derived during a maximal exercise is the maximum oxygen uptake (VO_2max). This is directly related to the amount of work performed. Predicted values vary slightly depending upon whether a cycle ergometer or treadmill is used, and calculated for the individual patient's height and age. A normal subject should reach 80% of their predicted value.

PATIENT 12.01

		Measured	Predicted	% predicted
Sex:	Male	Height (m):	1.67	
Age (yrs):	72	Weight (kg):	72	
Tobacco:	Non-smoker	BMI (kg/m²):	26	

	Measured	Predicted	% predicted
Maximum exercise performance:			
VO$_2$ (L/min)	1.21	1.72	68

In this subject VO$_2$max is low, so there is a problem somewhere. It could be breathing enough oxygen in, getting it across into the circulation or pumping it around to the muscles. There may also be a problem with the muscles themselves, or the subject may have quit because of pain somewhere or poor motivation. Looking at some additional parameters may give us a clue as to what is happening.

Ventilation

The maximum ventilation (VEmax, in L/min) achievable during exercise can be estimated by multiplying the FEV1 (in L) by a factor of 35. In a normal subject VEmax does not reach the predicted value, since ventilation is not usually the factor which limits exercise performance. VEmax should therefore be less than 80% of that predicted from FEV1. (The deficit between expected and observed VEmax is sometimes called the Breathing Reserve, which should be at least 15 L/min). Let's return to out patient with impaired exercise tolerance:

PATIENT 12.01

		Measured	Predicted	% predicted
Sex:	Male	Height (m):	1.67	
Age (yrs):	72	Weight (kg):	72	
Tobacco:	Non-smoker	BMI (kg/m²):	26	

	Measured	Predicted	% predicted
Maximum exercise performance:			
VO$_2$ (L/min)	1.21	1.72	68
VE (L/min)	61.8	58.8	105

Here VEmax exceeds the predicted value, which suggests that ventilation is the factor limiting exercise.

Heart rate

When ventilation is the cause of exercise limitation, the maximum heart rate will not reach 80% of the predicted value, as we can see in our previous example:

PATIENT 12.01

Sex:	Male	Height (m):	1.67		
Age (yrs):	72	Weight (kg):	72		
Tobacco:	Non-smoker	BMI (kg/m²):	26		
		Measured	*Predicted*	*% predicted*	
Maximum exercise performance:					
VO₂ (L/min)		1.21	1.72	68	
VE (L/min)		61.8	58.8	105	
Heart rate (bpm)		111	148	75	

Remember to check that the patient is not taking beta-blockers or other drugs which might impair the heart rate response before interpreting a low maximum value.

In a patient with a low VO_2max, if the heart rate reaches 80% of the predicted value, this suggests that circulatory factors are limiting exercise capacity:

PATIENT 12.02

Sex:	Male	Height (m):	1.86		
Age (yrs):	72	Weight (kg):	90		
Tobacco:	Non-smoker	BMI (kg/m²):	26		
		Measured	*Predicted*	*% predicted*	
Maximum exercise performance:					
VO₂ (L/min)		1.13	2.15	52	
VE (L/min)		36.4	90.6	40	
Heart rate (bpm)		141	148	95	

Notice that the maximum ventilation is well below predicted, indicating that ventilation is not a limiting factor. By "circulatory" I mean cardiac or pulmonary vascular.

Oxygen saturation is well maintained in normal subjects during exercise. If it falls then there is a ventilation-perfusion imbalance. This will occur in patients with airway or interstitial lung diseases, but also in pulmonary vascular problems such as pulmonary embolism. In patients with cardiac problems, desaturation is less common, so we can use this in a patient whose exercise test indicates a circulatory problem to decide whether it is the heart or the pulmonary vasculature that is responsible.

A patient who stops because of poor motivation will have a low VO_2max, and will achieve neither their predicted heart rate nor their predicted VEmax:

PATIENT 12.03

Sex:	Male	Height (m):	1.65
Age (yrs):	62	Weight (kg):	78
Tobacco:	Smoker	BMI (kg/m²):	29

	Measured	*Predicted*	*% predicted*
Maximum exercise performance:			
VO_2 (L/min)	1.27	2.16	59
VE (L/min)	58.2	86.1	68
Heart rate (bpm)	117	158	74

A similar picture may be seen in an unfit patient who is "deconditioned". This leads us on to the concept of the anaerobic threshold.

ANAEROBIC THRESHOLD

The validity of the concept of the Anaerobic Threshold (AT) and the derivation of it from exercise data, are the subjects of much debate. It is the cause of much confusion in those who do no more than think about exercise physiology all day, and mere mention of it can generate a glazed look. Much can be made of exercise data without reference to the AT. When we do use it, it is essential that you look to see where the computer has taken this point from: the most common method is to plot VO_2 against VCO_2 and look to see where the slope starts to increase.

At the AT, carbon dioxide production starts to increase faster than oxygen uptake. The reason for this is probably that lactate production has started to become significant, and this acid is buffered by combining with bicarbonate to produce CO_2 and water (figure 12.1).

AT should be greater than about 40% of the predicted VO_2max and is low if the muscles do not receive adequate oxygen (as in circulatory problems).

A common problem is patients whose exercise tolerance is impaired as a result of unfitness or deconditioning. The anaerobic threshold is low because the muscles are incapable of using the oxygen delivered to them, even though the supply is quite adequate. In lung disease, the anaerobic threshold is often not reached.

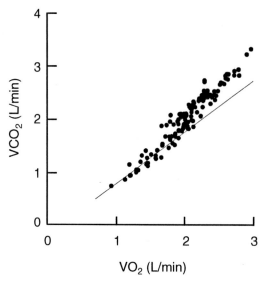

Figure 12.1

OTHER EXERCISE PARAMETERS

Introducing the concepts of the anaerobic threshold and starting to plot exercise parameters against each other leads us into deeper waters! There are quite a few other parameters which can be derived from exercise test data. For example, the pattern of breathing frequency and tidal volume change during exercise may give a clue as to whether a ventilatory problem is obstructive or restrictive. Muscular efficiency can be calculated as the oxygen consumption for work done. If arterial blood gases are sampled, dead space ventilation can be derived. These are all complex topics which I do not propose to cover: time for the specialist textbooks.

SUMMARY

☞   If VO_2 at maximum exercise is less than 80% predicted, exercise tolerance is impaired.

☞   If ventilation at maximum exercise is more than 80% of the predicted value, there is a ventilatory problem.

☞   If the heart rate at maximum exercise is more than 80% of the predicted value, there is a circulatory problem.

☞   Oxygen desaturation during exercise implies a problem with ventilation or the pulmonary circulation.

☞   The anaerobic threshold is less than 40% of the predicted VO_2max in circulatory problems or unfitness.

APPENDIX: WORKED EXAMPLES

So much for all the theory, now let's try and put it into practice. Here are some examples of patients referred to our laboratory for lung function testing recently. Come to your own conclusions, before turning the page to see if we agree. I have explained my reasoning in a short commentary after each patient.

EXAMPLE 1

Clinical information: Previously fit. Sudden onset of severe dyspnoea.

Sex:	Female	Height (m):	1.50
Age (yrs):	89	Weight (kg):	46
Tobacco:	Non-smoker	BMI (kg/m²):	20

	Measured	% Predicted	SR
Spirometry:			
FEV1 (L)	0.86	78	-0.64
VC (L)	1.27	87	-0.41
FEV1/VC (%)	68	94	-0.61
Lung Volumes: (Helium dilution)			
RV (L)	1.70	79	-1.25
FRC (L)	1.98	80	-0.94
TLC (L)	2.85	69	-2.15
Gas Transfer: (CO single breath, Hb=10.3 g/dl)			
TLCO (SI)	3.85	74	-1.13
KCO (SI)	1.72	136	+0.92

EXAMPLE 1

Report

Mild restrictive defect. This is unlikely to be the explanation of her shortness of breath, particularly since gas transfer is normal.

Commentary

Prediction equations are derived from populations which include only a very small number of 89 year olds, so all these results need to be interpreted with caution in this lady. Although the spirometry is normal, TLC takes precedence over VC in deciding about restriction, and the SR for TLC indicates that the problem is only mild. The anaemia could explain her shortness of breath, although the sudden onset might be a pulmonary embolism or even myocardial infarction. The message that we need to give is that further investigations are necessary, and the direction of these will be guided by clinical pointers and her general condition. We probably don't need to go as far as listing the causes of dyspnoea in our report.

EXAMPLE 2

Clinical information: Systemic lupus erythematosus, on prednisolone and azathioprine.

Sex:	Female	Height (m):	1.66
Age (yrs):	52	Weight (kg):	68
Tobacco:	Non-smoker	BMI (kg/m^2):	24

	Measured	% Pred	SR
Spirometry:			
FEV1 (L)	1.96	73	-1.84
VC (L)	2.64	84	-1.11
FEV1/VC (%)	74	93	-0.76
Lung Volumes: (Helium dilution)			
RV (L)	1.08	58	-2.17
FRC (L)	2.18	78	-1.19
TLC (L)	3.64	70	-2.58
Gas Transfer: (CO single breath, Hb=13.2 g/dl)			
TLCO (SI)	3.49	42	-4.11
KCO (SI)	1.07	66	-1.07

EXAMPLE 2

Report

Moderately severe restrictive defect with impaired gas transfer, consistent with pulmonary fibrosis.

Commentary

On spirometry we might be tempted to ignore the slightly low FEV1, given that VC and the FEV1/VC ratio are normal. However, when we proceed to look at full lung volumes there is indeed a restrictive defect. TLCO is low, indicating impaired gas transfer, but if this is the case why is the KCO normal ? The lungs are reduced in size, but if they were otherwise normal then the KCO should be greater than predicted; a normal KCO is consistent with impaired gas transfer. The most likely explanation is pulmonary fibrosis as a complication of her disease. Incidentally, if the KCO had been high we might have suggested that the clinician look for extra-pulmonary complications, such as pleural effusion or respiratory muscle weakness.

EXAMPLE 3

Clinical information: Sarcoidosis

Sex:	Male	Height (m):	1.81
Age (yrs):	37	Weight (kg):	115
Tobacco:	Non-smoker	BMI (kg/m^2):	35

	Measured	*% Predicted*	*SR*
Spirometry:			
FEV1 (L)	2.96	69	-2.56
VC (L)	4.62	90	-0.83
FEV1/VC (%)	64	79	-2.26
Lung Volumes: (Helium dilution)			
RV (L)	2.16	110	+0.48
FRC (L)	2.63	75	-1.42
TLC (L)	6.94	93	-0.64
Gas Transfer: (CO single breath, Hb=16.1 g/dl)			
TLCO (SI)	13.02	111	+0.96
KCO (SI)	1.84	116	+0.98

EXAMPLE 3

Report

Moderately severe obstructive defect, with normal gas transfer. This could be asthma or endobronchial sarcoidosis. Suggest serial peak flow monitoring and reversibility testing.

Commentary

The spirometry is a classical example of obstruction, which just falls into the "moderate" category on the basis of the SR for FEV1. In airflow obstruction we expect RV to be elevated; although greater than normal, it is still within the normal range, but on balance I don't think this indicates superimposed restriction in his case. Asthma is the most likely diagnosis, but we need to remind the clinician about the possibility of endobronchial inflammation and stenosis.

EXAMPLE 4

Clinical information: Incidental finding of high Hb. Is this primary or secondary polycythaemia ?

Sex:	Male	Height (m):	1.80
Age (yrs):	49	Weight (kg):	85
Tobacco:	Non-smoker	BMI (kg/m²):	27

	Measured	% Predicted	SR
Spirometry:			
FEV1 (L)	3.57	93	-0.50
VC (L)	4.33	90	-0.70
FEV1/VC (%)	82	105	
Lung Volumes: (Helium dilution)			
RV (L)	2.53	114	+0.78
FRC (L)	4.19	117	+1.04
TLC (L)	7.00	95	-0.44
Gas Transfer: (CO single breath, Hb=16.2 g/dl)			
TLCO (SI)	3.35	31	-5.21
KCO (SI)	0.59	40	-3.38

EXAMPLE 4

Report

Normal spirometry and lung volumes, but severe impairment of gas transfer. Assuming that the Hb is valid, this could be the result of a right-to-left shunt. Other possibilities include pulmonary vasculitis or an alveolar problem such as alveolar proteinosis. Suggest measurement of arterial blood gases, repeated after 30 mins on 100% oxygen if his PaO_2 on air is low. An echocardiogram or high resolution computerized tomography of the lungs might also be informative.

Commentary

The low gas transfer cannot be the result of fibrosis or emphysema, beacuse there is neither an obstructive nor a restrictive defect. Filling of alveoli by oedema fluid, inflammatory cells or other material can sometimes be seen with little interference with pulmonary mechanics. The clinical picture doesn't really fit with left ventricular failure, but he might have pneumocystis pneumonia or one of the rarities we discussed in Chapter 8, such a alveolar proteinosis. Pulmonary vasculitis is another possibility, and the polycythaemia points to the possibility of pulmonary oligaemia with a right-to-left shunt. (We do need to bear in mind that if his haemoglobin was low then the TLCO and KCO would be less abnormal, so it would be worth checking up on this before embarking on lots of other tests.)

EXAMPLE 5

Clinical information: Shortness of breath on exercise

	Measured	% Predicted	SR
Sex: Male Height (m): 1.67			
Age (yrs): 50 Weight (kg): 64			
Tobacco: Smoker BMI (kg/m²): 23			
Spirometry:			
FEV1 (L)	3.54	106	+0.38
VC (L)	4.53	113	+0.88
FEV1/VC (%)	76	97	-0.28
Lung Volumes: (Helium dilution)			
RV (L)	0.99	48	-2.60
FRC (L)	2.33	71	-1.59
TLC (L)	5.57	88	-1.00
Gas Transfer: (CO single breath, Hb=14.1 g/dl)			
TLCO (SI)	5.17	55	-2.86
KCO (SI)	0.97	65	-1.88

EXAMPLE 5

Report

Mild restrictive defect and low gas transfer compatible with early interstitial lung disease. Depending upon the chest radiographic appearances, high resolution computerized tomography of his lungs may be indicated.

Commentary

A restrictive defect can be diagnosed on the basis of a low RV, even when the VC and TLC are normal. Although the SR for RV indicates that this is moderately severe, I have called this mild because VC and TLC are so well preserved. Had the gas transfer been normal, we might have chosen to ignore the low RV, but these results suggest that he may well have early interstitial lung disease and warrants further investigation.

EXAMPLE 6

Clinical information: COAD

Sex:	Female	Height (m):	1.45
Age (yrs):	65	Weight (kg):	42
Tobacco:	Ex-smoker	BMI (kg/m²):	20

	Measured	*% Predicted*	*SR*	*After Salbutamol*
Spirometry:				
FEV1 (L)	0.54	35	-2.55	0.71
VC (L)	1.24	67	-1.41	1.61
FEV1/VC (%)	44	57	-5.00	
Lung Volumes: (Helium dilution)				
RV (L)	2.94	176	+3.68	
FRC (L)	3.51	151	+2.40	
TLC (L)	4.85	127	+1.79	
Gas Transfer: (CO single breath, Hb=14.6 g/dl)				
TLCO (SI)	2.91	48	-2.58	
KCO (SI)	0.84	53	-1.47	

EXAMPLE 6

Report

Moderately severe airflow obstruction with low gas transfer, suggesting the diagnosis of emphysema. No significant reversibility after salbutamol, but a longer therapeutic trial of bronchodilators may be warranted.

Commentary

The spirometry is obstructive, supported by the high RV. The low TLCO points to emphysema. Strictly speaking the KCO is still within normal limits as indicated by the SR, but at only 53% predicted it doesn't seem unreasonable to conclude that gas transfer is imparied. The increases in FEV1 and VC are both within the reproducibility of the tests, 0.2 and 0.45 L respectively, but the absence of significant reversibility in our laboratory should not deter the clinician from a longer therapeutic trial.

EXAMPLE 7

Clinical information: ? recurrent pulmonary embolism

Sex:	Female	Height (m):	1.70
Age (yrs):	62	Weight (kg):	85
Tobacco:	Non-smoker	BMI (kg/m²):	29

	Measured	*% Predicted*	*SR*
Spirometry:			
FEV1 (L)	1.77	68	-2.10
VC (L)	2.44	80	-1.38
FEV1/VC (%)	72	93	-0.76
Lung Volumes: (Helium dilution)			
RV (L)	1.55	74	-1.48
FRC (L)	2.12	73	-1.51
TLC (L)	3.67	67	-2.97
Gas Transfer: (CO single breath, Hb=12.2 g/dl)			
TLCO (SI)	7.08	86	-0.90
KCO (SI)	1.91	127	+0.82

EXAMPLE 7

Report

Moderately severe restrictive defect. Although extensive pulmonary infarction can cause restriction, the normal gas transfer makes this explanation of the low TLC unlikely. Could the depth of inspiration have been limited by pleuritic pain, or is there evidence of pleural effusion or any other cause of extrapulmonary restriction ?

Commentary

A we have seen in earlier examples, a low FEV1 with normal VC might be ignored, but would probably indicate the need for full lung volumes to be measured. Restriction is usually only seen in severe pulmonary embolic disease, in which case gas transfer would be reduced. Although within normal limits, the KCO is greater than predicted, so it is more likely that her lungs are normal but inadequately inflated.

EXAMPLE 8

Clinical information: Diffuse lung shadowing on CXR

Sex:	Male	Height (m):	1.67
Age (yrs):	68	Weight (kg):	47
Tobacco:	Smoker	BMI (kg/m²):	17

	Measured	*% Predicted*	*SR*
Spirometry:			
FEV1 (L)	1.90	69	-1.59
VC (L)	2.68	76	-1.37
FEV1/VC (%)	71	94	-0.57
Lung Volumes: (Helium dilution)			
RV (L)	4.60	186	+5.15
FRC (L)	4.69	136	+2.11
TLC (L)	6.35	101	-0.11
Gas Transfer: (CO single breath, Hb=14.6 g/dl)			
TLCO (SI)	1.02	12	-4.95
KCO (SI)	0.26	20	-3.84

EXAMPLE 8

Report

Mixed restrictive/obstructive picture. Low gas transfer could be explained by either emphysema or pulmonary fibrosis, or a combination of both. High resolution computerized tomography of his lungs might help in assessing the relative contribution of these two processes.

Commentary

There are a number of causes of an elevated RV, but the extrapulmonary ones such as expiratory muscle weakness and skeletal problems are excluded by the low gas transfer. Such a high RV is suggestive of airway collapse, but if this is the case then something else must be going for him to maintain a normal FEV1/VC ratio. The most likely explanation is that he has two diseases, for example emphsema and fibrosing alveolitis. The clinician, with the patient and his scans in front of them, is going to be in a better position than us to decide what is going on.

EXAMPLE 9

Clinical information: Rheumatoid arthritis, short of breath

Sex:	Female	Height (m):	1.65
Age (yrs):	74	Weight (kg):	64
Tobacco:	Non-smoker	BMI (kg/m²):	24

	Measured	% Predicted	SR
Spirometry:			
FEV1 (L)	0.96	46	-2.92
VC (L)	2.24	89	-0.60
FEV1/VC (%)	43	45	-3.46
Lung Volumes: (Helium dilution)			
RV (L)	3.52	162	+3.91
FRC (L)	4.08	147	+2.64
TLC (L)	5.89	115	+1.31
Gas Transfer: (CO single breath, Hb=11.5 g/dl)			
TLCO (SI)	4.25	59	-2.47
KCO (SI)	1.00	71	-0.80

EXAMPLE 9

Report

Moderately severe obstructive defect with impaired gas transfer. Does she have bronchiolitis obliterans ?

Commentary

The spirometry and high RV are classical of obstruction. The TLC is not particularly high, but this is a poor indicator of superimposed restriction when measured by Hlium dilution. The low TLCO suggests emphysema, but why is the KCO normal ? Rheumatoid arthritis can be associated with this pattern of a low TLCO and normal KCO, for reasons that are unclear. In the presence of obstruction, we obviously need to consider bronchiolitis as a complication of her rheumatoid.

EXAMPLE 10

Clinical information: Basal crackles, poor left ventricular function on echo, little improvement with diuretics.

Sex:	Male	Height (m):	1.67
Age (yrs):	72	Weight (kg):	76
Tobacco:	Non-smoker	BMI (kg/m²):	28

	Measured	*% Predicted*	*SR*
Spirometry:			
FEV1 (L)	1.68	64	-1.82
VC (L)	1.87	54	-2.50
FEV1/VC (%)	90	121	+2.28
Lung Volumes: (Helium dilution)			
RV (L)	0.99	38	-3.73
FRC (L)	1.47	42	-3.36
TLC (L)	2.94	46	-4.79
Gas Transfer: (CO single breath, Hb=14.8 g/dl)			
TLCO (SI)	3.07	39	-3.33
KCO (SI)	1.39	112	+0.56
Maximum Exercise Performance: (Cycle ergometer)			
VO2 (L/min)	1.21	68	
VE (L/min)	61.8	105	
Heart rate (bpm)	111	75	

EXAMPLE 10

Report

Severe restrictive defect with impaired gas transfer. Exercise is appears to be limited by ventilatory rather than circulatory factors. This picture is more suggestive of pulmonary fibrosis than left ventricular failure.

Commentary

The spirometry and lung volumes are typical of a restrictive problem. As we have already seen, the KCO would be high if the lungs were this small because of extra-pulmonary factors, so the low TLCO and normal KCO are both compatible with impaired gas exchange. An exercise test was requested to try and sort out whether his lungs or his left ventricle were the main problem, and the fact that he reaches the predicted ventilation without achieving 80% of the predicted maximum heart rate suggests that his lungs are the main problem. The crackles may be fibrosis rather than oedema.

EXAMPLE 11

Clinical information: Previous hemi-thyroidectomy. "Wheeze" on exercise.

Sex:	Male	Height (m):	1.85
Age (yrs):	63	Weight (kg):	105
Tobacco:	Non-smoker	BMI (kg/m²):	31

	Measured	*% Predicted*	*SR*
Spirometry:			
FEV1 (L)	3.68	101	+0.07
VC (L)	5.78	123	+1.78
FEV1/VC (%)	64	84	-1.71
Lung Volumes: (Helium dilution)			
RV (L)	3.93	152	+3.29
FRC (L)	4.30	112	+0.83
TLC (L)	9.31	120	+2.30
Gas Transfer: (CO single breath, Hb=14.2 g/dl)			
TLCO (SI)	12.9	124	+1.77
KCO (SI)	1.56	115	+0.79

Flow Volume Loop:

EXAMPLE 11

Report

Mild airflow obstruction with elevated TLCO consistent with a diagnosis of asthma. No evidence of an upper airway problem on the flow-volume loop.

COMMENTARY

In an asymptomatic individual, the slightly low FEV1/VC ratio could have been ignored: the FEV1 is fine and the low ratio reflects the supra-normal VC. However, his wheeze prompted further investigation and full lung volumes show a very high RV. This suggests that he does indeed have airflow obstruction, and with an elevated TLCO asthma seems the most likely diagnosis. The shape of his flow-volume loop does not suggest tracheal compression by his residual thyroid tissue.

IN CONCLUSION......

I hope these examples give you some idea of lung function interpretation in clinical practice. It is a skill which comes with practice, and part of the art of writing reports on data such as these is deciding what to leave in and what to leave out. Obviously this is quite a subjective matter, and every individual has their own style.

SUMMARY

☞   Check the anthropometric data and consider how applicable prediction equations are to that individual.

☞   Don't overinterpret isolated or mild abnormalities.

☞   Use any clinical information you have to decide whether the lung function test results fit with the provisional diagnosis.

☞   Suggest other possible diagnoses for the clinician to consider.

☞   Recommend further tests if you think they would be helpful.

BIBLIOGRAPHY

PHYSIOLOGY

Pulmonary pathophysiology - the essentials. West JB. Williams and Wilkins, Baltimore 1992. ISBN 0-683-08936-0

Respiratory physiology - the essentials. West JB. Williams and Wilkins, Baltimore 1995. ISBN 0-683-08937-4

Applied respiratory physiology. Nunn JF. Butterworths. London 1987. ISBN 0-407-00342-8

LUNG FUNCTION TESTS

Classic texts:

Clinical tests of respiratory function. Gibson GJ. Chapman and Hall, London 1996. ISBN 0-412-56890-X

Lung function. Cotes J. Blackwell, Oxford 1993. ISBN 0-632-03526-9

Other smaller books:

Pulmonary function testing. A practical approach. Wanger J. Williams and Wilkins, Baltimore 1992. ISBN 0-683-17834-2

Pulmonary function testing. Principles and practice. Conrad SA, Kinasewitz GT, Gearage RB. Churchill Livingstone, New York 1984. ISBN 0-443-08182-4

Pulmonary function testing. Cherniak RM. WB Saunders, Philadelphia 1992. ISBN 0-7216-4014-1

Manual of pulmonary function testing. Ruppell G. Mosby, St Louis 1994. ISBN 0-8016-7789-0

Pulmonary function: a guide for clinicians. Laszlo G. Cambridge University Press, Cambridge 1994. ISBN 0-521-44679-1.

LUNG FUNCTION IN DISEASE

Respiratory function in disease. Bates DV. WB Saunders, Philadelphia 1989. ISBN 0-7216-1592-9

Clinical tests of respiratory function. Gibson GJ. Chapman and Hall, London 1996. ISBN 0-412-56890-X

INDEX

Printed in the United Kingdom
by Lightning Source UK Ltd.
107269UKS00002B/1-76